CANCER DIET FOR KIDS

Eating to Fight Cancer: A Nutritious Guide for Kids with Cancer

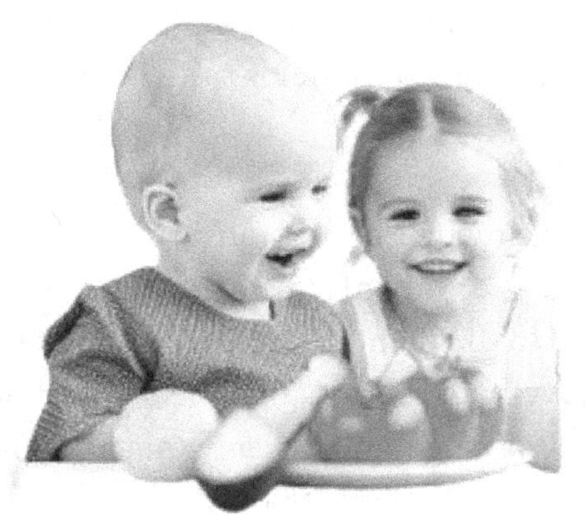

BETTIE J.STEWART

TABLE OF CONTENTS

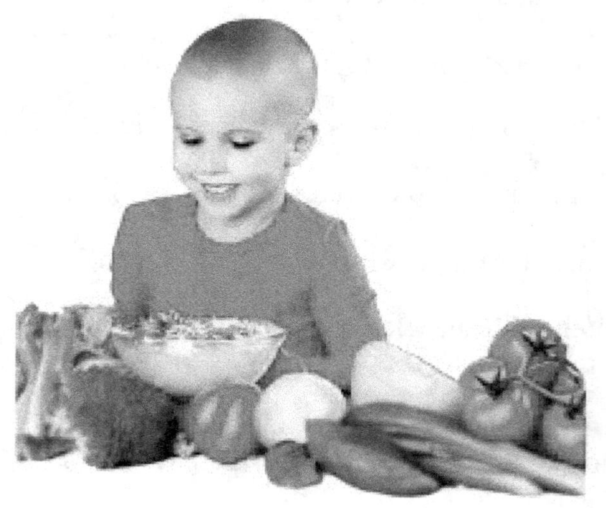

INTRODUCTION TO CANCER DIETS FOR KID

My daughter was diagnosed with a rare form of cancer when she was just three years old. We were devastated and felt helpless. But then we stumbled across a cookbook that contained recipes specifically designed for people with cancer. After doing some research, we found out that these recipes were designed to help fight cancer and boost the body's natural healing processes.

We immediately got started with the recipes, and soon my daughter was eating a nutritious, cancer-fighting diet. The recipes were simple and easy to follow, and the ingredients were easy to find. We also made sure to avoid any foods that could potentially be bad for her health.

Within a few months, my daughter's condition had improved dramatically. Her energy levels increased, her pain had decreased, and her tumors had shrunk.

After a year of following the cancer-fighting diet, my daughter was declared cancer-free.

We were amazed at the power of food and nutrition. We were so thankful for the cookbook that had helped us make this journey. We are now firm believers in the power of healthy eating, and we continue to cook healthy meals for our family every day. That specific cookbook's main takeaway has been embedded within this cookbook to help your loved ones in reversing their cancer conditions.

Cancer is one of the most common diseases found in children and adolescents. While there is no single diet that can prevent or cure cancer, there are certain dietary practices that can help reduce the risk of developing cancer, as well as improve the quality of life for those who have already been diagnosed.

In this book, we will explore the evidence-based nutrition strategies that can help children and adolescents with cancer in a variety of ways. We will discuss the importance of healthy eating habits, the benefits of nutrient-dense foods, and the potential risks of certain dietary choices. Additionally, we will cover meal planning, food safety, and strategies to help children stick to their diets.

By the end of this book, you should have a comprehensive understanding of how to make healthy dietary choices for your child or adolescent with cancer. You will be equipped with the knowledge and resources to help your child or adolescent maintain a healthy weight, get the proper nutrition, and make food choices that support their overall wellbeing.

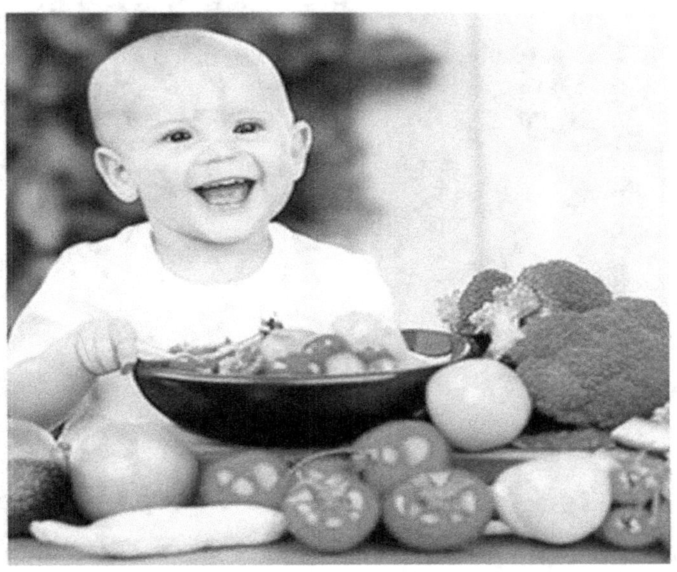

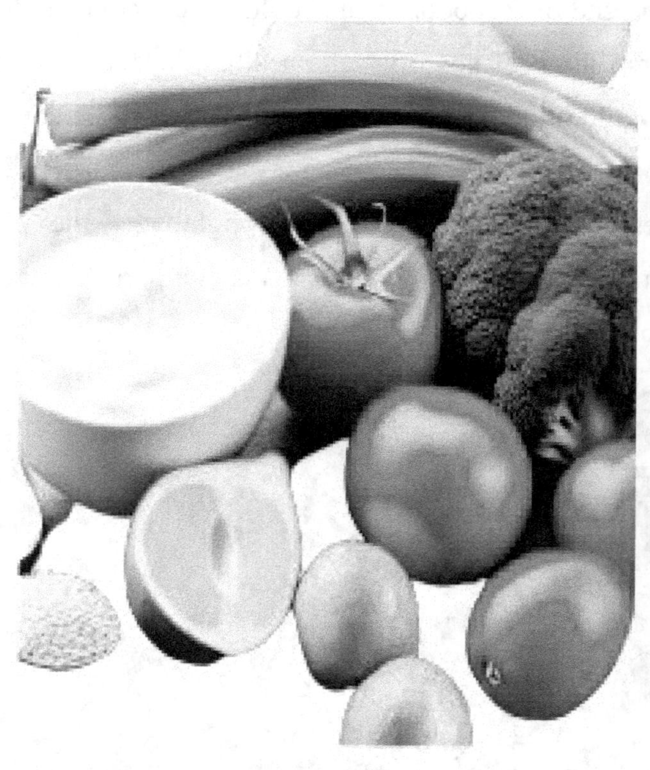

CHAPTER 1: UNDERSTANDING THE BASICS OF CANCER DIETS

Cancer is a serious disease that can have a significant impact on a person's life. Diet and nutrition can play an important role in managing cancer and its symptoms. A cancer diet consists of foods that are beneficial to the body and may support the body's natural healing processes.

Eating a balanced diet that includes plenty of fruits, vegetables, and whole grains can help the body to fight off cancer, while avoiding processed food, refined sugars, and unhealthy fats can help to reduce the risk of cancer.

Furthermore, the American Cancer Society recommends that cancer survivors follow the Dietary Guidelines for Americans, which recommends eating a variety of nutrient-dense foods, such as plenty of fruits and vegetables, as well as whole grains, lean proteins, and healthy fats.

Additionally, it's important to stay hydrated and limit alcohol consumption. Eating a balanced diet can help reduce the risk of cancer recurrence and improve overall health.

By following a well-balanced diet, cancer survivors can reduce their risk of cancer recurrence and improve their overall health.

Determining the Right Diet

The right cancer diet will depend on a patient's individual needs, so it's important for them to discuss their dietary choices with a doctor or nutritionist. In some cases, a doctor may recommend a specific diet for a particular type of cancer or to help reduce the risk of recurrence. For example, a doctor may recommend a low-fat diet for people with breast cancer or a low glycemic index diet for people with pancreatic cancer.

Foods to Eat

A cancer diet should focus on eating plenty of fruits and vegetables, lean protein sources, whole grains, and healthy fats. Additionally, it is important to focus on eating nutrient-dense foods that are high in antioxidants, vitamins, and minerals.

Fruits and Vegetables

Eating plenty of fruits and vegetables is essential for a healthy diet, and especially for those fighting cancer. Fruits and vegetables are rich in vitamins, minerals, antioxidants, and fibre, which can help to fight off disease and support the immune system. Eating a variety of colourful fruits and vegetables can provide a wide array of essential nutrients.

Protein

Lean proteins such as fish, skinless poultry, beans, and tofu can provide essential nutrients and help to increase satiety. Eating a variety of different proteins can help to ensure that the body is getting all the essential amino acids.

Whole Grains

Whole grains are a great source of fibre, B vitamins, and antioxidants. Eating whole grains can help to regulate blood sugar levels and keep the digestive system healthy.

Healthy Fats

Healthy fats such as olive oil, nuts, and avocados are a great way to get essential fatty acids and can help to increase satiety. Fats can also help to absorb fat-soluble vitamins from other foods.

Foods to Avoid

In addition to eating healthy foods, it is important to avoid processed foods, refined sugars, and unhealthy fats. Processed foods often contain preservatives, additives, and unhealthy fats that can be harmful to the body. Refined sugars can cause a spike in blood sugar levels and can lead to weight gain. Unhealthy fats, such as trans fats, can increase the risk of heart disease and should be avoided.

Drinks

It is important to stay hydrated when fighting cancer, so drinking plenty of water is essential. Additionally, avoiding sugary beverages and drinking unsweetened tea and coffee can help to provide essential antioxidants and nutrients.

Observation

Eating a healthy diet is essential for those fighting cancer, as it can help to support the body's natural healing processes and fight off disease. Eating plenty of fruits, vegetables, and whole grains while avoiding processed food, refined sugars, and unhealthy fats can help to reduce the risk of cancer and its symptoms. Additionally, staying hydrated and drinking unsweetened beverages can help to keep the body healthy.

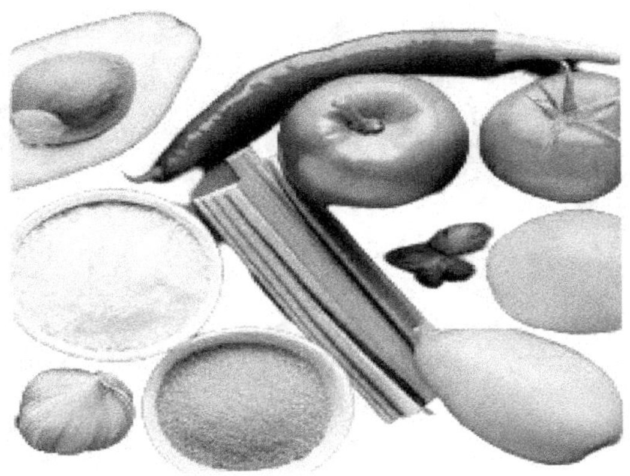

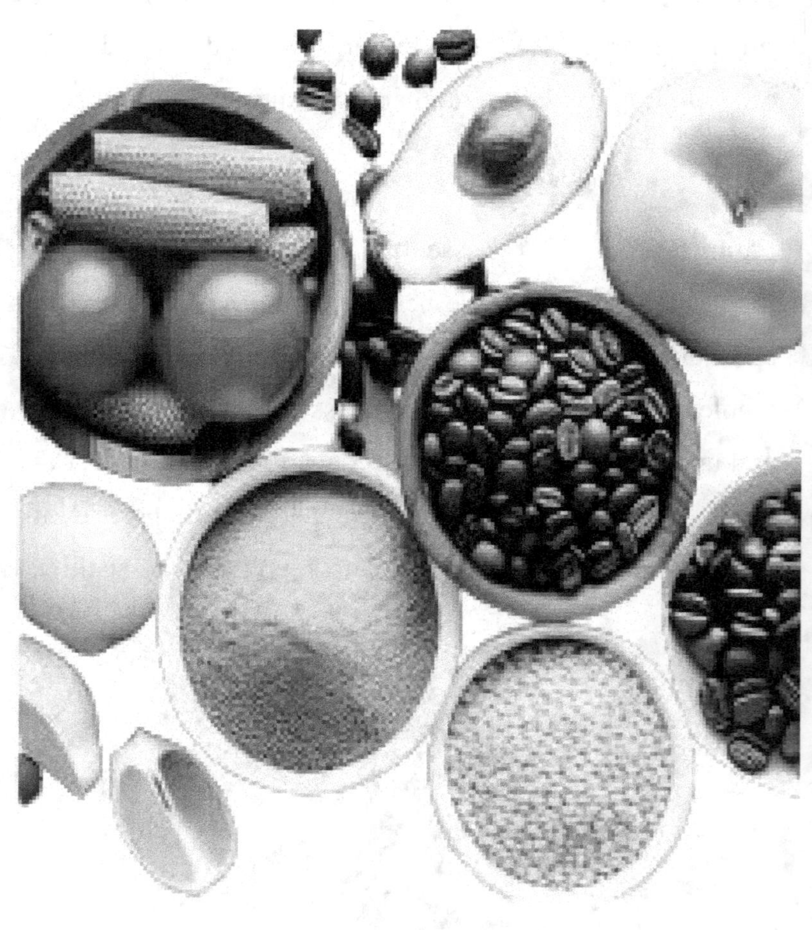

Chapter 2: Food Choices for Kids with Cancer

Food choices for kids with cancer should be tailored to meet their individual needs. Generally, a balanced diet with plenty of fruits, vegetables, whole grains, lean proteins, and dairy products is recommended. As with any child, limiting junk food and sugary drinks is important. Additionally, providing plenty of fluids and snacks throughout the day can help ensure adequate nutrition. It is also important to consider food safety when preparing meals for a child with cancer, as their weakened immune system can make them more vulnerable to food-borne illnesses.

Special nutritional needs may be necessary for certain cancer treatments, such as chemotherapy and radiation, as well as for certain medical conditions related to the cancer diagnosis. In such cases, it may be necessary to consult with a dietitian to determine the best food choices for the child.

The nutritional options for youngsters with cancer may be overwhelming and confusing. With so many various meals and nutrition regimens out there, it may be tough to know what is best for a kid with cancer. The purpose of this chapter is to offer parents with information regarding food choices for kids with cancer, including what sorts of foods are most useful and how to make healthy diet choices.

Benefits of Eating a Healthy Diet

Eating a nutritious, balanced diet is crucial for any kid, but it may be particularly critical for children with cancer. Eating well may bring a multitude of advantages, including:

❖ Strengthening the immune system: A balanced diet may assist to enhance the immune system and make it easier for the body to fight cancer.

❖ Improving nutrition: Eating a balanced diet may assist to ensure that a kid is receiving all the vital vitamins and minerals they need to be healthy.

❖ Supporting therapies: Eating a nutritious diet may assist to support treatments like as chemotherapy and radiation therapy, as well as lower the risk of adverse effects from these treatments.

Types of Foods for Kids with Cancer

When picking meals for a kid with cancer, it is crucial to choose ones that are nutrient-dense and rich in key vitamins and minerals. Some of the greatest sorts of meals for a kid with cancer include:

❖ Fruits and veggies: Fruits and vegetables are filled with vitamins and minerals and are a fantastic way to receive fibre, antioxidants, and other critical nutrients.

❖ Protein: Protein is vital for mending cells and tissue and helping to develop the immune system. Good sources of protein include lean meats, seafood, eggs, nuts, and legumes.

❖ Whole grains: Whole grains are an excellent source of carbs, fiber, and other nutrients, and may assist to deliver sustained energy.

❖ Healthy fats: Healthy fats, such as olive oil, canola oil, and avocados, are crucial for delivering needed fatty acids and helping to boost the immune system.

Tips for Making Healthy Food Choices

When it comes to selecting good dietary choices for kids with cancer, there are some basic guidelines that may assist. These include:

❖ Focus on fresh: Fresh fruits and vegetables are a terrific method to receive critical vitamins and minerals.

❖ Avoid processed foods: Processed foods are generally heavy in sugar, fat, and salt, and may be damaging to a child's health.

❖ Think outside the box: Try to introduce different foods to your youngster and be creative with meals.

❖ Make meals fun: Get your youngster involved in the preparation process and make meals interesting and pleasurable.

❖ Plan ahead: Planning meals ahead of time will assist to ensure that your kid is receiving a balanced diet.

Observation

Making appropriate eating choices for kids with cancer is vital for preserving their health and supporting their therapies. Eating a balanced diet that includes fresh fruits and vegetables, lean meats, whole grains, and healthy fats will assist to ensure that a kid is receiving all the critical nutrients they need. With the correct dietary plan, parents can assist their kid with cancer to be healthy and strong.

Chapter 3: What Foods to Avoid

Kids with cancer should avoid meals that are heavy in fat, especially saturated fats, as well as those with added sweets and high amounts of salt. These meals may lead to an unhealthy weight gain, which can raise the chance of acquiring additional conditions and make treatment more difficult. Additionally, certain unhealthy diets, such as processed meats and fried foods, might include substances that can raise the risk of cancer and interfere with therapy.

High fat meals such as fast food, processed snacks, and fried foods should be avoided. These meals are often heavy in saturated fats, which may raise the risk of developing additional conditions and make treatment more difficult. Additionally, these meals might also lead to an unhealthy weight increase.

Foods with added sugars should also be avoided. Consuming too much sugar may lead to obesity, which raises the chance of acquiring additional ailments. Additionally, sugar may interfere with the body's capacity to metabolize vital nutrients, making it more difficult for children with cancer to acquire the nourishment they need.

Foods heavy in salt should also be avoided. Consuming too much salt may lead to elevated blood pressure, which can interfere with therapy. Additionally, excessive salt diets might add to dehydration, a typical adverse effect of cancer therapy.

In summary, kids with cancer should avoid high fat diets, foods with added sugars, and foods rich in salt. These foods may lead to an unhealthy weight gain, raise the risk of developing other illnesses, interfere with therapy, and make it more difficult for children with cancer to acquire the nourishment they need.

The frequent adverse effects of such eating include higher chance of acquiring other illnesses, interference with cancer therapy and difficulty for the body to absorb important nutrients.

When it comes to the diets of children with cancer, there are certain foods that should be avoided. These foods can negatively affect their health and may even interfere with their treatment.

1. Processed Foods:

Processed foods are full of additives and preservatives, which can be hard to digest and can cause inflammation in the body. Processed foods can also be high in sugar, salt, and unhealthy fats, which can be dangerous for children with cancer.

2. Refined Grains:

Refined grains have had most of their nutritional value stripped away during the refining process. White bread, white rice, and pasta are all examples of refined grains. These foods are high in carbohydrates and can cause blood sugar levels to spike, which can be dangerous for children with cancer.

3. Fried and High-Fat Foods:

Fried and high-fat foods are often high in unhealthy fats that can increase inflammation in the body. These foods can also be difficult to digest and can cause nausea and other digestive issues in children with cancer.

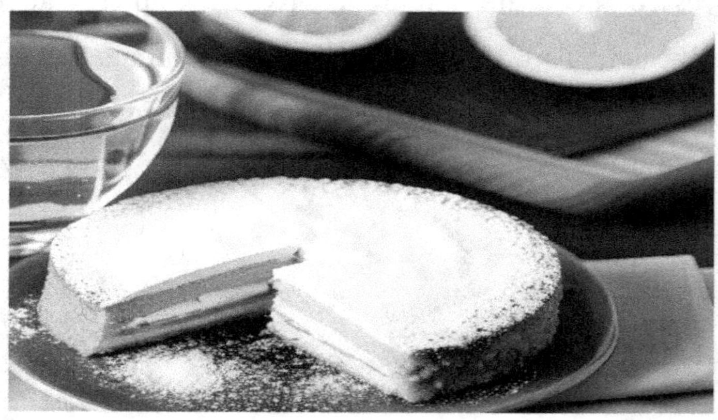

4. High-Sugar Foods:

Highly processed and high-sugar foods such as candy, cakes, cookies, and sodas are all bad for children with cancer. High-sugar foods can cause blood sugar levels to spike and can cause inflammation in the body.

5. Alcohol:

Alcohol can interfere with treatments and can weaken a child's immune system. It can also cause digestive issues, dehydration, and fatigue.

6. Caffeinated Beverages:

Caffeine is a stimulant that can interfere with treatments, weaken a child's immune system, and increase anxiety.

7. Raw or Undercooked Foods:

Raw or undercooked foods can increase the risk of food poisoning and can be difficult to digest.

It is important for children with cancer to follow a healthy, balanced diet that includes whole grains, fruits and vegetables, lean proteins, and healthy fats. Eating a variety of foods can provide them with the nutrients they need to help them stay healthy and fight their disease.

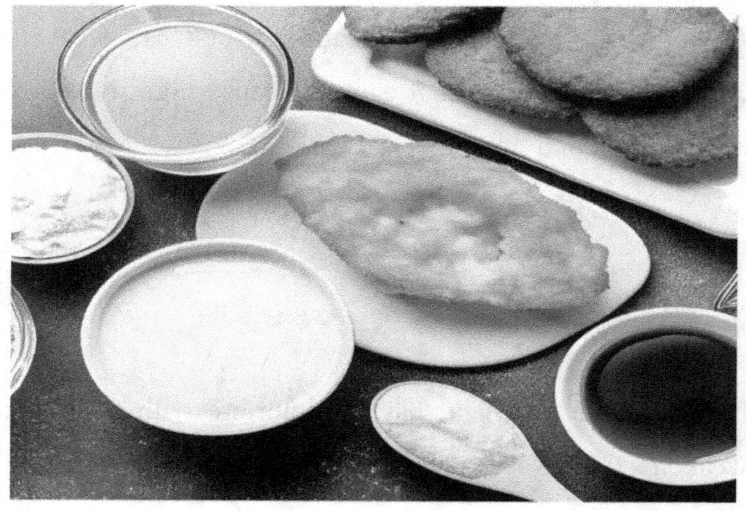

Chapter 4: Healthy Food Alternatives for Kids with Cancer

Kids with cancer should eat healthy foods instead of unhealthy foods for a number of reasons. The first reason is that healthy foods provide important nutrients, vitamins, minerals and fiber that can help the body stay strong during treatment. Healthy foods can also help boost the immune system and provide additional energy to help the body fight off infections and other illnesses.

Unhealthy foods, on the other hand, can be detrimental to a cancer patient's health. Unhealthy foods are often high in calories and unhealthy fats and contain very little of the essential nutrients that cancer patients need to stay healthy. Additionally, unhealthy foods can add to the side effects of cancer treatment, such as nausea, vomiting and constipation, making it difficult for the patient to stay nourished.

Finally, healthy foods can help to maintain a healthy weight, which is important for cancer patients, as they are often at risk of becoming malnourished or underweight due to their illness.

A balanced diet of healthy foods can help to ensure that the patient is getting the necessary nutrients while also maintaining a healthy weight.

Healthy food alternatives for kids living with cancer are important to support their health and wellbeing. Eating healthy foods is essential for giving the body the energy and nutrients it needs to stay strong and cope with the effects of cancer treatment.

1. Focus on plant-based proteins:

Plant-based proteins such as beans, legumes, and tofu can provide a healthy alternative to animal proteins. They are also rich in fibre, vitamins and minerals. Adding these two meals or snacks can help increase the nutrient value while still providing a delicious meal.

2. Include fresh fruits and vegetables:

Fresh fruits and vegetables are packed with vitamins, minerals, and antioxidants. Eating a variety of different fruits and vegetables can help to ensure a balanced diet and provide the nutrients necessary for a healthy body.

3. Choose healthy fats:

Healthy fats such as olive oil, avocados, nuts, and seeds are a great way to add flavour and nutrition to meals. These fats provide essential fatty acids and can help to keep the body running efficiently.

4. Eat whole grains:

Whole grains such as whole wheat bread, brown rice, quinoa, and oats are a great source of complex carbohydrates. Eating these foods can help to provide energy and help to keep the body.

5. Limit processed and sugary foods:

Processed and sugary foods can be tempting but are not healthy alternatives. They are often high in sugar and contain very little in terms of nutrition. Limiting these foods can help to ensure that kids are getting the nutrients they need.

These are just a few healthy food alternatives for kids living with cancer. Eating a balanced diet and limiting processed and sugary foods can help to ensure that kids are getting the nutrition they need to stay strong and healthy.

It is also important to talk to a doctor or nutritionist to make sure that the food choices are safe and appropriate for the individual's needs.

Chapter 5: Meal Planning for Kids with Cancer

Meal preparation for a kid with cancer may be a challenging chore. Not only is it crucial to ensure that the kid is getting appropriate nourishment, but it is also important to consider the child's individual requirements and preferences. In addition, it is crucial to adapt meal plans as the child's demands and therapies change.

The first step in meal planning for a kid with cancer is to evaluate the child's nutritional requirements. This may be done by communicating with the child's healthcare team, including the oncologist, dietician, and/or nurse. A licensed dietitian may give recommendations on the child's unique nutritional needs, including calorie and nutrient requirements, as well as additional factors such as food allergies. The nutritionist may also propose particular meal planning tactics, such as including nutrient-dense meals and snacks into the child's diet.

The next stage is to establish a meal plan that matches the child's nutritional requirements while also addressing the child's likes and dislikes. It is crucial to provide meals that the youngster loves, since this might assist encourage the child to eat. Additionally, it is crucial to incorporate a range of meals to ensure that the youngster is eating a balanced diet. It is also important to plan meals ahead of time, since this may make meal preparation simpler and more effective.

When preparing meals for a child with cancer, it is crucial to consider the youngster's appetite and energy levels. Some children may have lower appetites and energy levels owing to the adverse effects of treatments, so it is crucial to include meals that are simple to digest and give appropriate nourishment. Additionally, meals should be changed as the child's requirements and therapies vary. For example, the dietician may propose increasing the quantity of protein in the diet if the kid is having weight loss or muscle wasting.

Finally, it is crucial to include the youngster in meal planning. This may make the youngster feel more in charge of their nutrition and may help enhance the child's appetite and interest in eating. The youngster may assist pick foods, organize meals, and even participate with meal preparation.

Meal planning for a child with cancer may be tough, but with the correct advice and participation of the kid, it is possible to construct meals that offer enough nutrition while also taking into consideration the child's individual requirements and preferences.

By following these suggestions, parents and caregivers may help ensure that their child with cancer is getting the nutrition they need to be healthy throughout treatment.

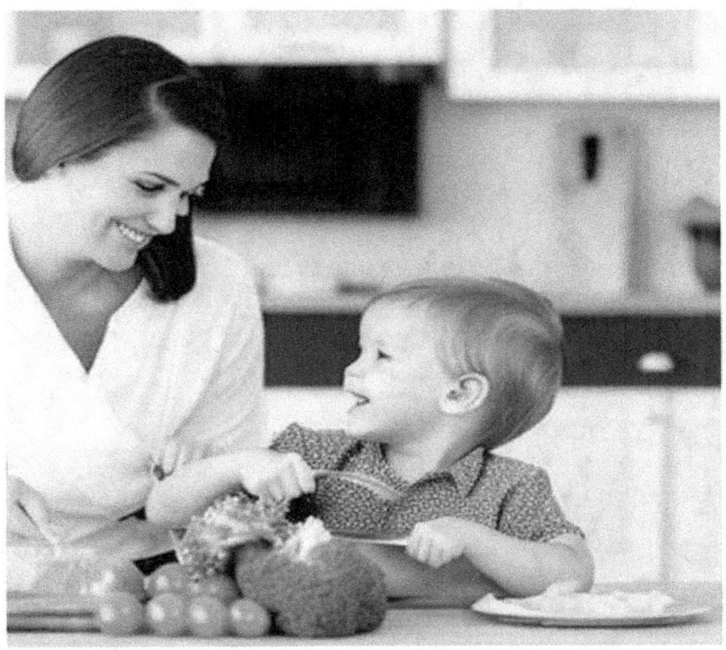

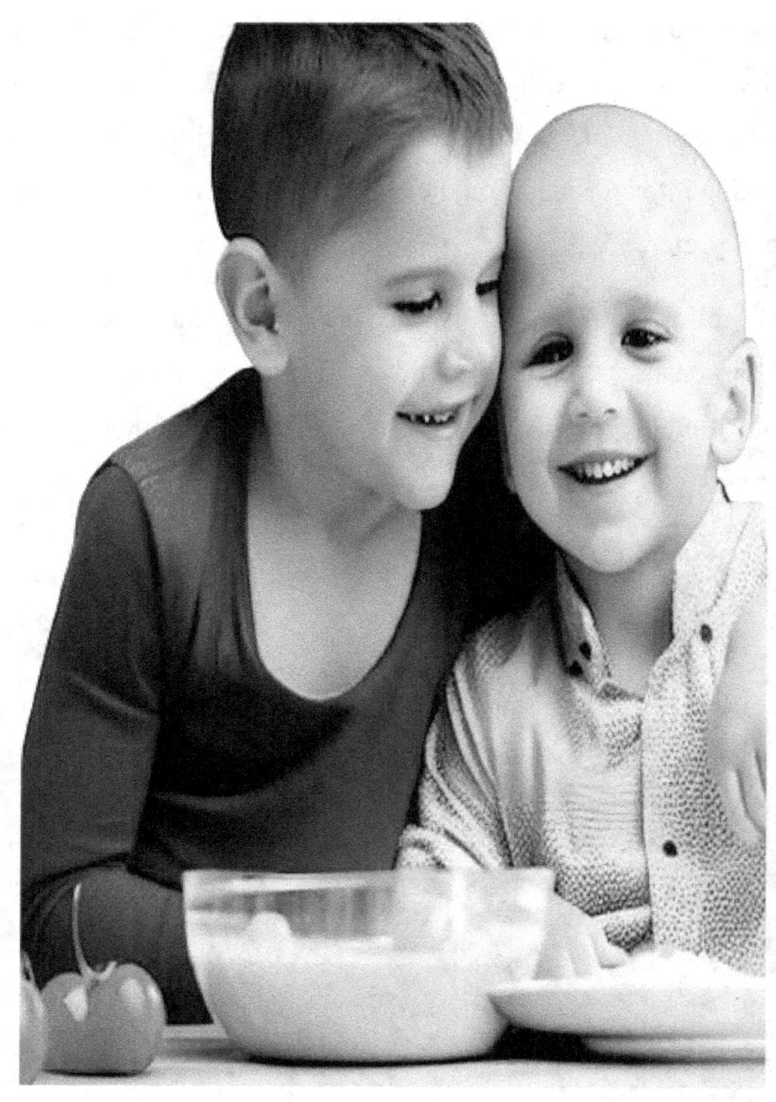

Chapter 6: Recipes for Kids with Cancer

This chapter is about recipes for children with cancer. It provides an in-depth look at how to create meals that are both nutritious and delicious for kids with cancer. The recipes in this chapter are designed to be simple and easy to prepare, while still providing the essential nutrients needed for children with cancer. Additionally, this chapter focuses on using ingredients that are easy to find and cost-effective, as well as providing tips for making the recipes fun and enjoyable for the child.

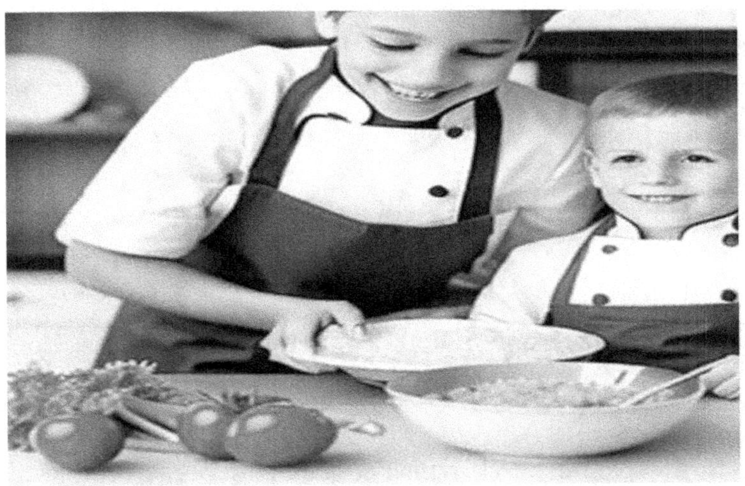

Breakfast

1.Vegetable Omelette

Ingredients:

- ❖ 2 eggs
- ❖ 1/4 cup onion, diced
- ❖ 1/4 cup bell pepper, diced
- ❖ 1/4 cup mushroom, diced
- ❖ 1 tablespoon olive oil
- ❖ Salt and pepper, to taste
- ❖

Instructions:

1. Heat the olive oil in a medium-sized skillet over medium heat.

2. Add the diced onion, bell pepper, and mushrooms. Cook until vegetables are softened, about 5 minutes.

3. In a separate bowl, whisk together the eggs until well-combined.

4. Pour the egg mixture over the vegetables and season with salt and pepper.

5. Cook until the eggs are set, about 3 minutes. Flip the omelette and cook for an additional 2 minutes.

6. Remove from heat and serve warm. Enjoy!

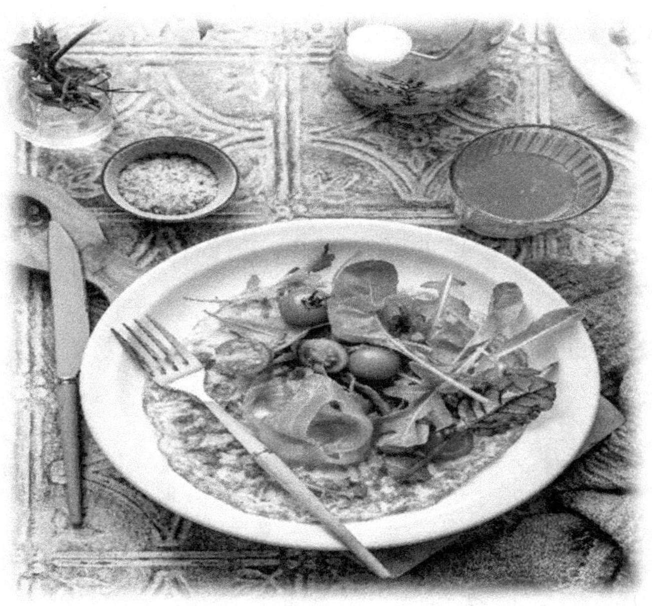

2. Banana Oat Pancakes

Ingredients:

- ❖ 1 cup rolled oats.
- ❖ 1 ripe banana
- ❖ 1 cup almond milk
- ❖ 1 teaspoon baking powder
- ❖ 1 teaspoon ground cinnamon
- ❖ 1/4 teaspoon salt
- ❖ 1 tablespoon coconut oil
- ❖ Non-stick cooking spray

Instructions:

1. In a blender, blend together the oats, banana, almond milk, baking powder, cinnamon, and salt until smooth.

2. Heat a non-stick skillet or griddle over medium heat and lightly coat with coconut oil and non-stick cooking spray.

3. Pour the batter onto the skillet or griddle and cook until the edges begin to dry and bubbles form on the surface.

4. Flip and cook the other side until golden brown.

5. Serve warm with your favorite toppings such as honey, blueberries, or sliced bananas. Enjoy!

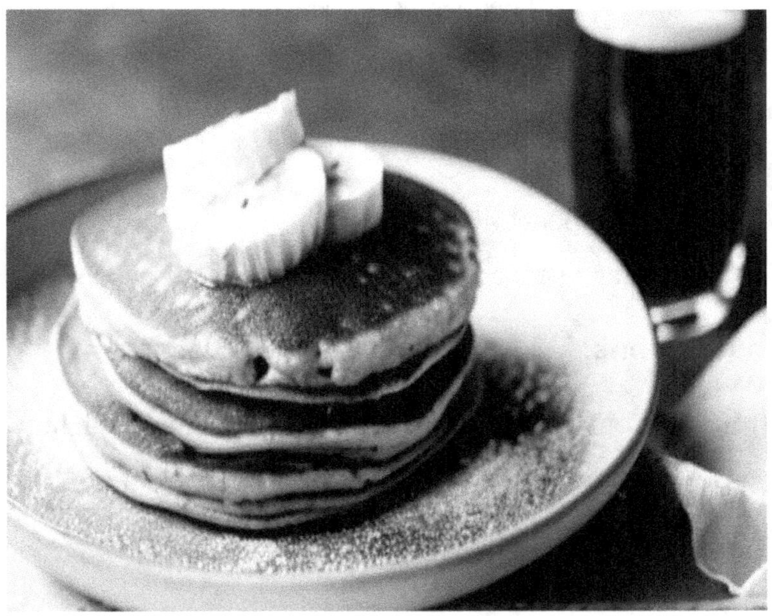

3. Breakfast Burrito Bowl

Ingredients:

- ❖ 1 cup cooked white rice.
- ❖ 1 cup cooked black beans.
- ❖ 1 cup cooked chicken, chopped.
- ❖ 1/2 cup bell peppers, chopped.
- ❖ 1/2 cup onion, chopped.
- ❖ 1/4 cup shredded cheese.
- ❖ 1/4 cup salsa
- ❖ 1 tablespoon olive oil
- ❖ Salt and pepper to taste.

Instructions:

1. Heat the olive oil in a large skillet over medium-high heat.

2. Once the oil is hot, add the onions and bell peppers. Cook until the vegetables are softened, about 5 minutes.

3. Add the cooked chicken, beans, and rice to the skillet. Stir to combine.

4. Add the salsa, salt, and pepper, stirring to combine.

5. Cook for an additional 5 minutes, stirring occasionally.

6. Remove the skillet from the heat and stir in the shredded cheese.

7. Serve the burrito bowl in individual bowls, topped with additional salsa and cheese, if desired. Enjoy!

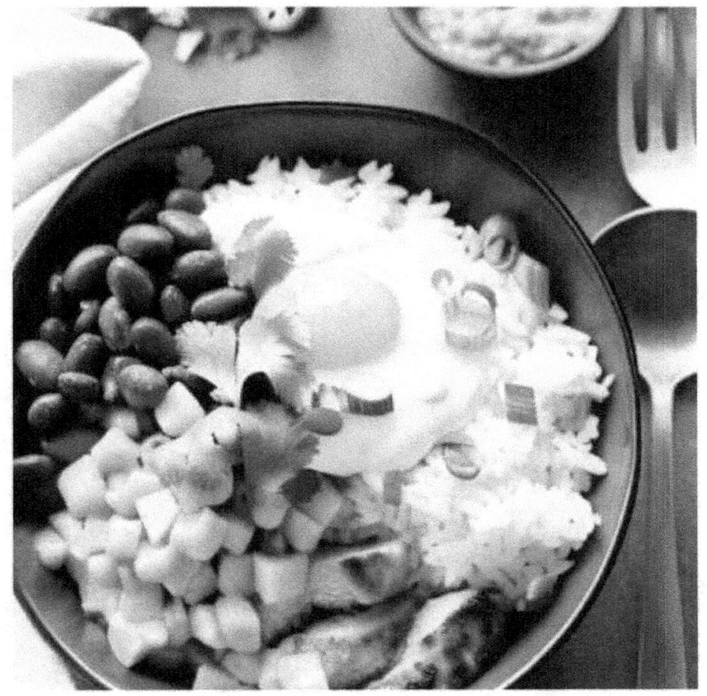

4.   Chocolate Chip Pancakes

Ingredients:

* 1 cup all-purpose flour
* 2 tablespoons white sugar
* 2 teaspoons baking powder
* 1/2 teaspoon salt
* 1 tablespoon vegetable oil
* 1 egg
* 3/4 cup milk
* 1/2 cup semi-sweet chocolate chips
* Butter

Instructions:

1. In a medium bowl, whisk together flour, sugar, baking powder, and salt.

2. In a separate bowl, whisk together vegetable oil, egg, and milk.

3. Add wet ingredients to dry ingredients and mix until just combined.

4. Add chocolate chips and stir until evenly distributed.

5. Heat a large skillet over medium heat and add a pat of butter.

6. Once the butter is melted, scoop 1/4 cup of batter onto the skillet.

7. Cook for 1-2 minutes until the edges start to look dry.

8. Flip the pancake and cook for an additional 1-2 minutes.

9. Repeat with remaining batter.

10. Serve pancakes with butter and syrup. Enjoy!

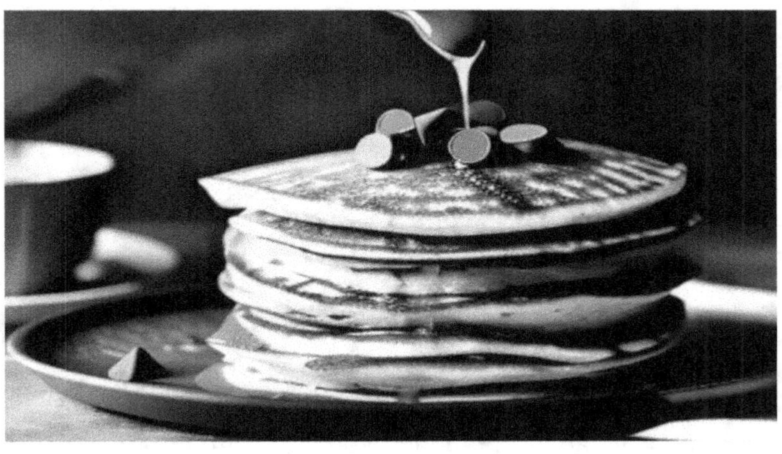

5. Cheesy Egg and Veggie Breakfast Quesadillas

Ingredients:

- ❖ 2 large eggs
- ❖ 2 tablespoons of vegetable oil
- ❖ 1/4 cup of diced onion
- ❖ 1/4 cup of diced bell peppers
- ❖ 1/4 cup of diced mushrooms
- ❖ 1/4 cup of diced cooked ham
- ❖ 2 tablespoons of chopped fresh chives
- ❖ 1/2 cup of shredded cheddar cheese
- ❖ 2 large whole-wheat tortillas
- ❖ Salt and pepper, to taste

Instructions:

1. Heat the vegetable oil in a large skillet over medium heat.

2. Add the onions, peppers, mushrooms, and ham and cook until the vegetables are tender, about 3-4 minutes.

3. Add the eggs and scramble until cooked through.

4. Add the chives and season with salt and pepper to taste.

5. Divide the egg mixture and spread it evenly over the tortillas.

6. Sprinkle the cheese on top of the eggs and fold the tortillas in half.

7. Carefully transfer the quesadillas to the skillet and cook until the bottom is golden brown, about 3 minutes.

8. Flip the quesadillas and cook until the other side is golden brown, about 3 minutes.

9. Cut the quesadillas into wedges and serve warm. Enjoy!

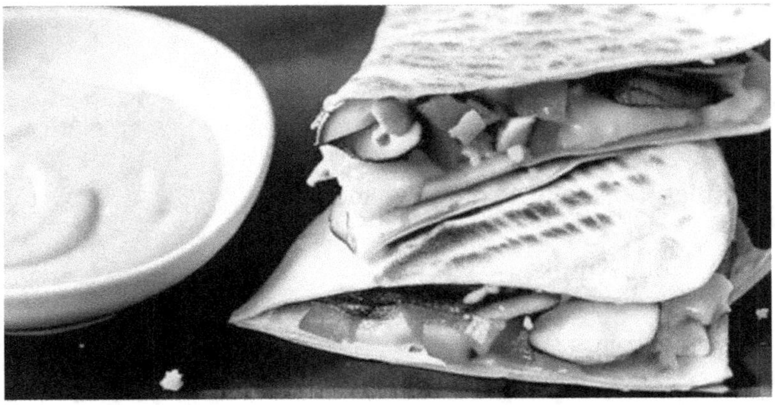

6. Gingerbread Waffles with Fruit

Ingredients:

-2 cups all-purpose flour

-2 teaspoons baking powder

-1 teaspoon baking soda

-1 teaspoon ground ginger

-1 teaspoon ground cinnamon

-1/4 teaspoon ground nutmeg

-Pinch of salt

-2 eggs

-2 tablespoons unsalted butter, melted

-2 cups buttermilk

-1/4 cup molasses

-1/4 cup packed light brown sugar

-Assorted fresh fruit such as blueberries, raspberries, and banana slices

Instructions:

1. Preheat a waffle iron according to manufacturer's instructions.

2. In a large bowl, whisk together the flour, baking powder, baking soda, ginger, cinnamon, nutmeg, and salt.

3. In a medium bowl, whisk together the eggs, butter, buttermilk, molasses, and brown sugar until blended.

4. Slowly pour the wet ingredients into the dry ingredients and whisk until just combined.

5. Lightly grease the preheated waffle iron. Pour the batter onto the iron, filling it about three-quarters full. Close the iron and cook for about 3 minutes, or until the waffles are golden brown and cooked through.

6. Serve the hot waffles with fresh fruit and maple syrup, if desired. Enjoy!

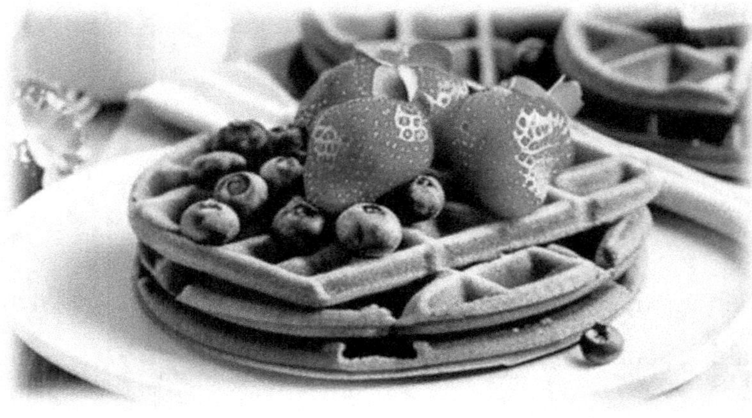

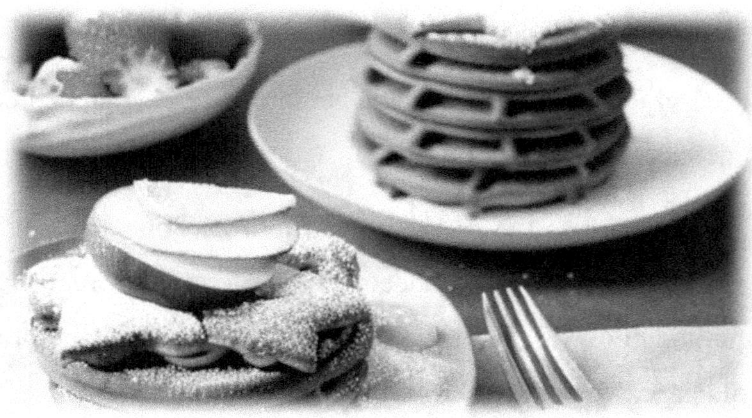

7. Fruity Oatmeal with Berries:

Ingredients:

1 cup rolled oats

1 cup milk (or milk alternative such as almond milk)

2 tablespoons honey

1 tablespoon chia seeds

½ teaspoon ground cinnamon

1 cup mixed berries (such as blueberries, raspberries, and blackberries)

Instructions:

1. In a medium saucepan, combine the rolled oats, milk, honey, chia seeds, and ground cinnamon.

2. Place the saucepan over medium heat and bring to a boil, stirring regularly.

3. Reduce the heat to low and simmer for about 5 minutes, or until the oats are tender.

4. Remove the saucepan from the heat, stir in the mixed berries, and let sit for a few minutes.

5. Serve the fruity oatmeal warm with a dollop of plain yogurt, if desired. Enjoy!

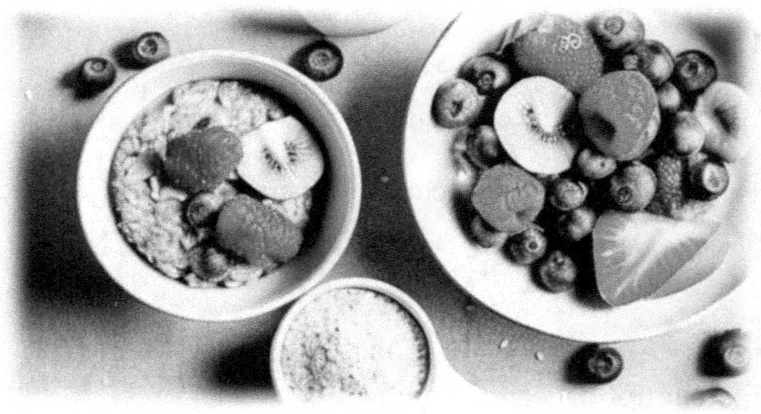

8. Vegetable Frittata

Ingredients:

- 2 tablespoons olive oil

- 1/2 cup diced onion

- 1/2 cup diced bell pepper

- 1/2 cup diced zucchini

- 1/2 cup diced mushrooms

- 1/2 cup frozen spinach, thawed and drained

- 6 eggs

- 1/4 cup grated Parmesan cheese

- Salt and pepper to taste

Instructions:

1. Preheat oven to 350 degrees F.

2. Heat olive oil in a large skillet over medium heat. Add the onion, bell pepper, zucchini, mushrooms, and spinach and cook until vegetables are softened, about 5 minutes.

3. In a large bowl, whisk together the eggs, Parmesan cheese, salt, and pepper.

4. Pour the egg mixture into the skillet with the vegetables and cook until the edges are set, about 5 minutes.

5. Transfer the skillet to the preheated oven and bake until the frittata is set and golden brown, about 15 minutes.

6. Serve warm and enjoy!

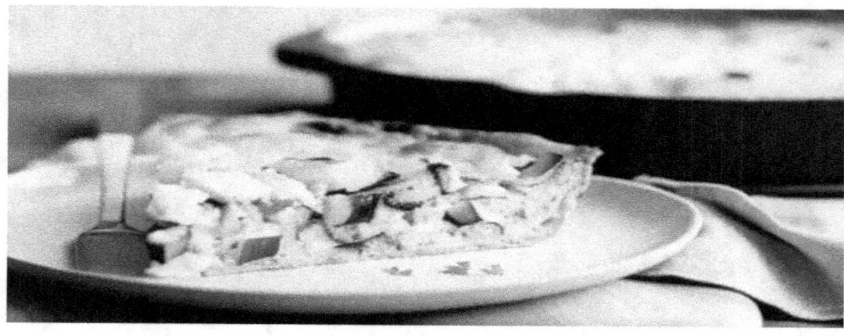

9. Breakfast Egg Cups

Ingredients:

- 4 large eggs

- 1/4 cup of cooked bacon, diced

- 1/4 cup of diced bell peppers

- 1/4 cup of shredded cheddar cheese

- Salt and pepper to taste

Instructions:

1. Preheat your oven to 375°F.

2. Grease a muffin tin with nonstick cooking spray or butter.

3. Crack one egg into each muffin cup.

4. Top each egg with equal amounts of bacon, bell peppers and cheese.

5. Season with salt and pepper.

6. Bake for 15 to 20 minutes or until eggs are cooked through and the cheese is golden brown.

7. Let cool slightly before serving. Enjoy!

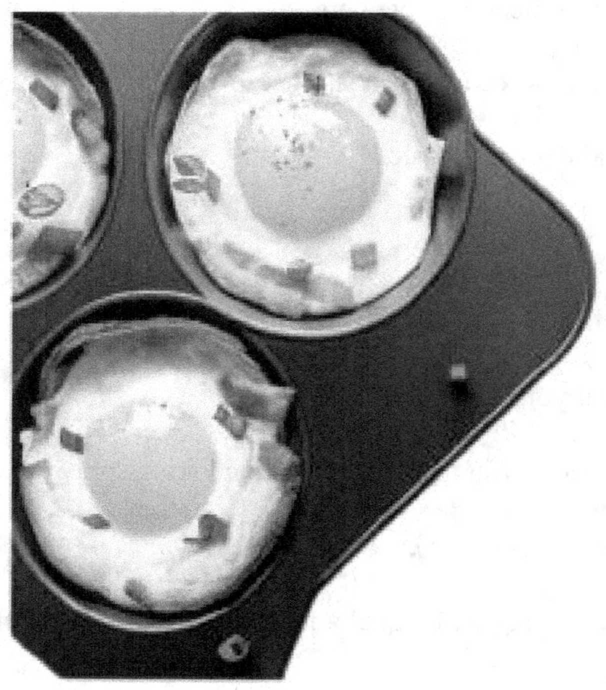

10. Breakfast Recipe for Kids with Cancer:

Ingredients:

-1 cup of rolled oats

-1/4 cup of raisins

-2 tablespoons of honey

-1/4 cup of almond milk

-1 banana, thinly sliced

-1 teaspoon of cinnamon

-1/4 cup of blueberries

-1 tablespoon of coconut oil

Instructions:

1. In a medium-sized bowl, combine the rolled oats, raisins, honey, and almond milk.

2. Heat a large skillet over medium heat and add the banana slices.

3. Sprinkle the cinnamon over the banana slices and let cook until the bananas are lightly browned, about 5 minutes.

4. Add the oat mixture to the skillet and cook until the oats are lightly browned, about 10 minutes.

5. Add the blueberries and coconut oil and stir until everything is combined.

6. Serve warm. Enjoy!

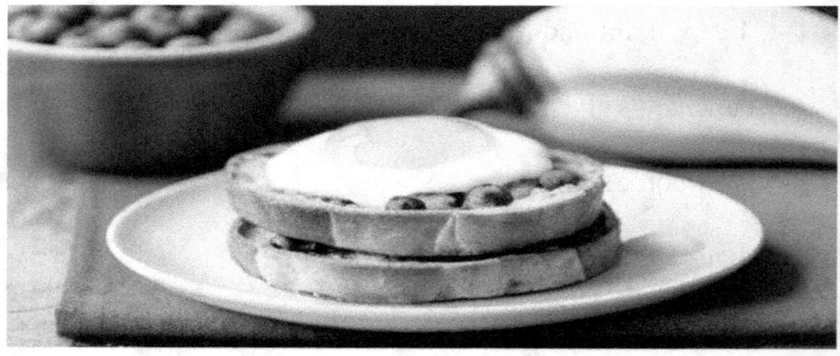

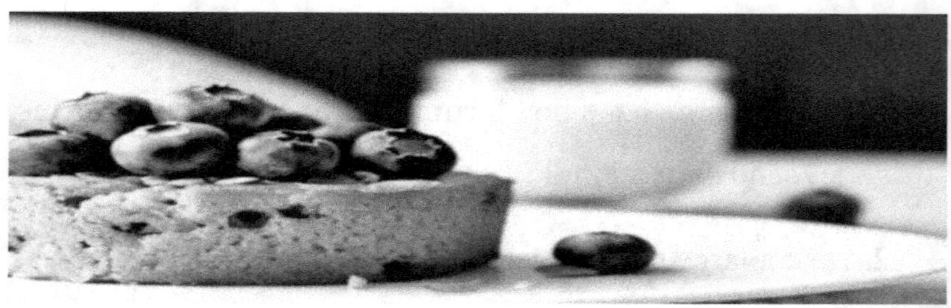

Lunch

Welcome to the lunch section for kids with cancer! Eating the right food can help children with cancer stay strong and healthy during their treatment, and the recipes in this section are designed to provide the nutrition they need. All of the recipes are easy to make and full of flavor, so that children can still enjoy their meals. Eating the right food can also make a huge difference in their recovery. So let's get started!

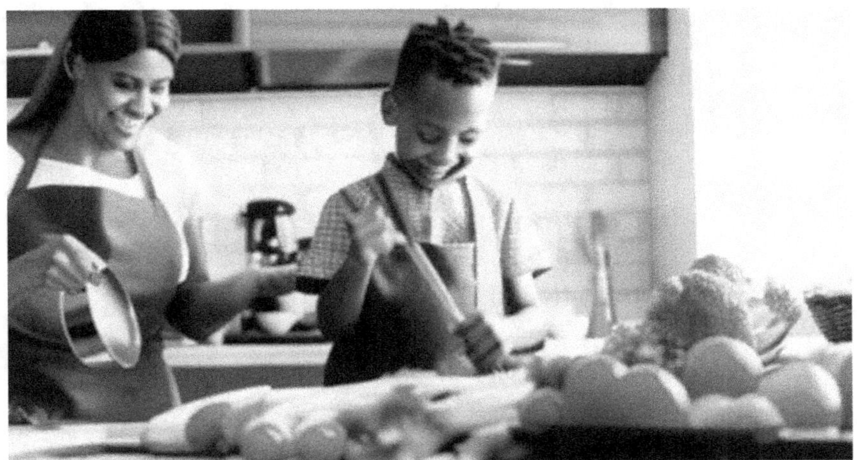

1. Veggie Salad Wrap:

Ingredients:

- 2 whole wheat tortillas

- ½ cup of cooked quinoa

- 1 cup of cooked mixed vegetables (such as broccoli, cauliflower, carrots, etc)

- ½ cup of cooked beans

- 2 tablespoons of olive oil

- Salt and pepper to taste

Instructions:

1. Preheat oven to 350°F.

2. Place the tortillas on a baking sheet and bake for 8-10 minutes.

3. In a medium bowl, mix together the cooked quinoa, cooked mixed vegetables, and cooked beans.

4. Drizzle the olive oil over the mixture and season with salt and pepper to taste.

5. Divide the mixture and place it in the center of each tortilla.

6. Fold the sides of the tortilla in, and then roll the tortilla up.

7. Cut each wrap in half and serve.

Enjoy!

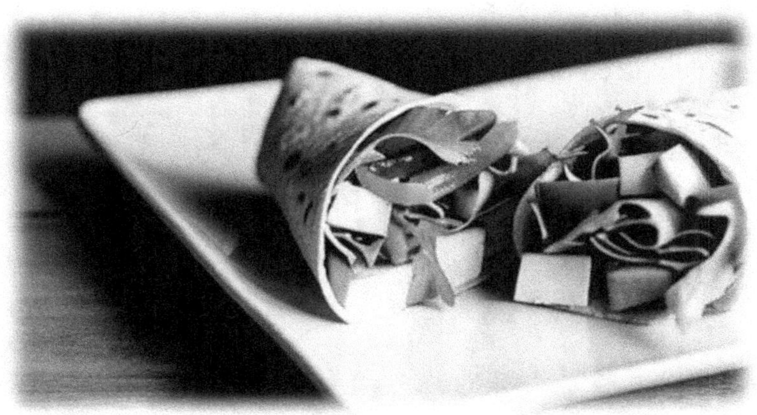

2. Vegetarian Rice Bowl

Ingredients:

-1 cup cooked brown rice

-1/2 cup cooked black beans

-1/4 cup diced bell peppers

-1/4 cup diced carrots

-1/4 cup corn

-1/4 cup diced avocado

-1/4 cup diced tomatoes

-1/4 cup cooked mushrooms

-1 tablespoon olive oil

-1 tablespoon lime juice

-Salt and pepper to taste

Instructions:

1. Heat the olive oil in a large skillet over medium heat.

2. Add the bell peppers, carrots, corn, mushrooms, and cook until the vegetables are tender.

3. Add the cooked brown rice, black beans, and cook until heated through.

4. Add the diced tomatoes, avocado, and lime juice, and cook until heated through.

5. Season with salt and pepper to taste.

6. Divide the rice bowl among four plates and serve. Enjoy!

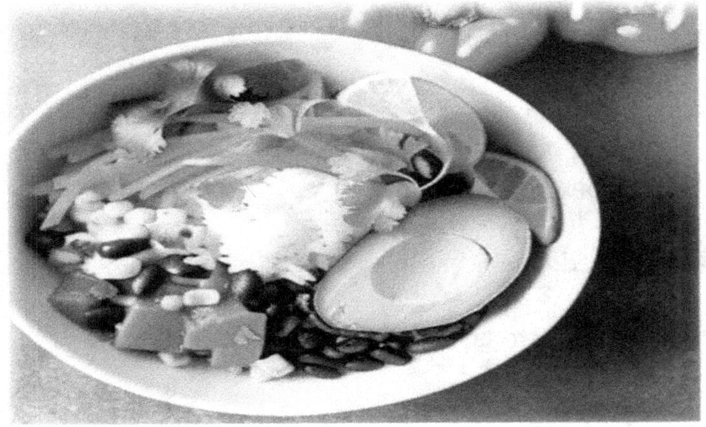

3. Vegetable Stuffed Peppers:

Ingredients:

-4 large bell peppers, any color

-1/2 cup cooked brown rice

-1/2 cup cooked black beans

-1/2 cup diced tomatoes

-1 teaspoon chili powder

-1/2 teaspoon garlic powder

-1/4 teaspoon cumin

-1/4 teaspoon oregano

-1/4 cup shredded cheese

-Salt and pepper to taste

Instructions:

1. Preheat the oven to 350 degrees F.

2. Cut the peppers in half and remove the seeds and stems. Place on a baking sheet.

3. In a large bowl, mix together the cooked rice, black beans, tomatoes, chili powder, garlic powder, cumin, oregano, salt, and pepper.

4. Stuff each pepper half with the mixture and top with the shredded cheese.

5. Bake for 20 minutes, or until the peppers are tender.

6. Serve warm with a side of your favorite veggies. Enjoy!

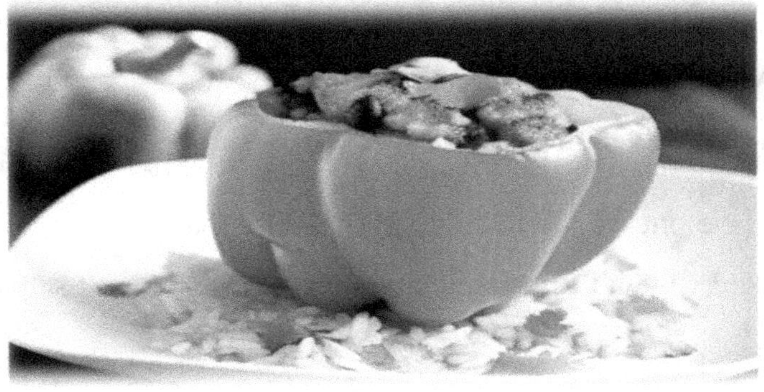

4.Vegetable Quesadilla:

Ingredients:

-1 tablespoon olive oil

2-3 cups of chopped vegetables of choice (such as bell peppers, onions, mushrooms, and spinach)

-2 whole wheat tortillas

-1/4 cup of grated cheese (low-fat, if desired)

- Salt and pepper, to taste

Instructions:

1. Heat olive oil in a large skillet over medium heat.

2. Add the chopped vegetables and cook for 3-4 minutes, or until the vegetables are softened.

3. Place one of the tortillas in the skillet, and top with the cooked vegetables, grated cheese, and a sprinkle of salt and pepper.

4. Place the second tortilla on top, and cook for 3-4 minutes, or until the bottom tortilla is lightly browned.

5. Flip the quesadilla over and cook for an additional 3-4 minutes, or until the second side is lightly browned.

6. Cut into wedges and serve warm. Enjoy!

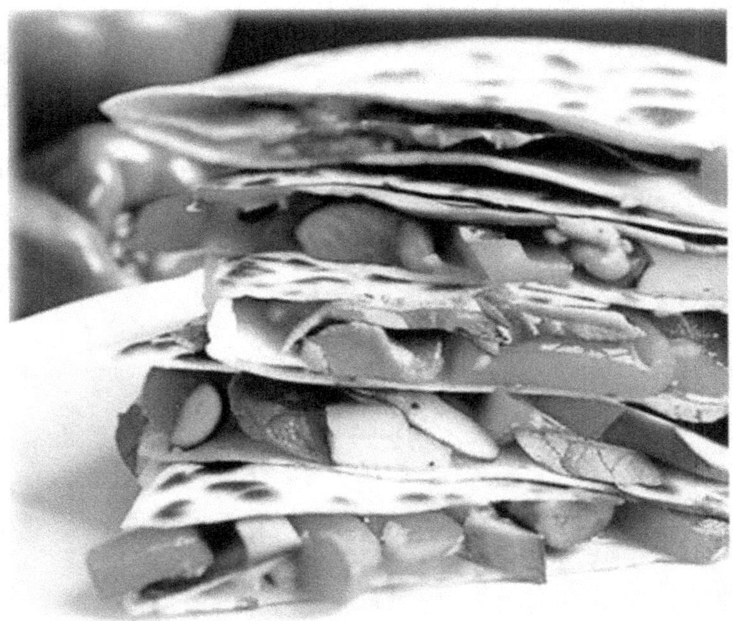

5.Veggie-Stuffed Chicken:

Ingredients:

-2 boneless, skinless chicken breasts

-1/4 cup of diced bell peppers

-1/4 cup of diced mushrooms

-1/4 cup of diced zucchini

-1/2 cup of cooked quinoa

-1/4 cup of grated Parmesan cheese

-1/4 cup of low-sodium chicken broth

-1 tablespoon of olive oil

-Fresh herbs of your choice, such as oregano, thyme, and basil

-Salt and pepper to taste

Instructions:

1. Preheat oven to 375 degrees Fahrenheit.

2. Heat the olive oil in a skillet over medium heat.

3. Add the diced bell peppers, mushrooms, and zucchini and sauté until lightly browned and tender, about 5 minutes.

4. Stir in the cooked quinoa and Parmesan cheese and cook for another 2 minutes.

5. Remove from heat and season with salt, pepper, and herbs of your choice.

6. Place the chicken breasts on a cutting board and use a sharp knife to cut a pocket into the side of each breast.

7. Stuff each chicken breast with the vegetable-quinoa mixture and place in a baking dish.

8. Pour the chicken broth into the dish and cover with aluminum foil.

9. Bake for 30-35 minutes, or until the internal temperature of the chicken reaches 165 degrees Fahrenheit.

10. Serve warm with a side of your favorite vegetables. Enjoy!

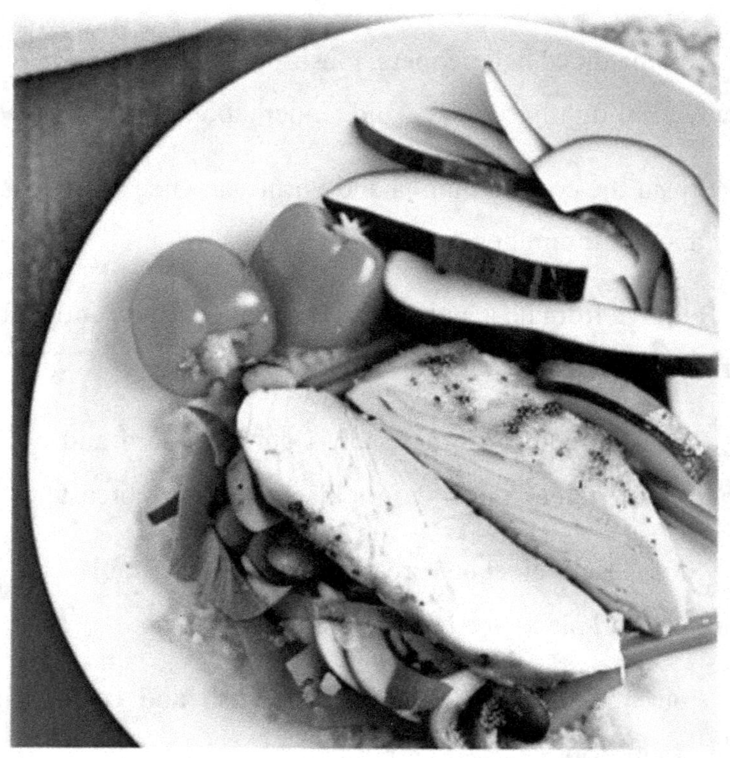

6.Grilled Cheese and Veggie Sandwich:

Ingredients:

-2 slices of whole wheat bread

-2 slices of American cheese

-1/4 cup of thinly sliced bell peppers

-1/4 cup of thinly sliced cucumbers

-2 tablespoons of butter

Instructions:

1. Heat a skillet or griddle over medium heat.

2. Spread butter on one side of each slice of bread.

3. Place one slice of bread in the skillet, butter side down.

4. Layer the cheese and veggies on the bread.

5. Place the other slice of bread on top, butter side up.

6. Cook until bread is golden brown and cheese is melted.

7. Flip the sandwich and cook until the other side is golden brown.

8. Serve warm and enjoy!

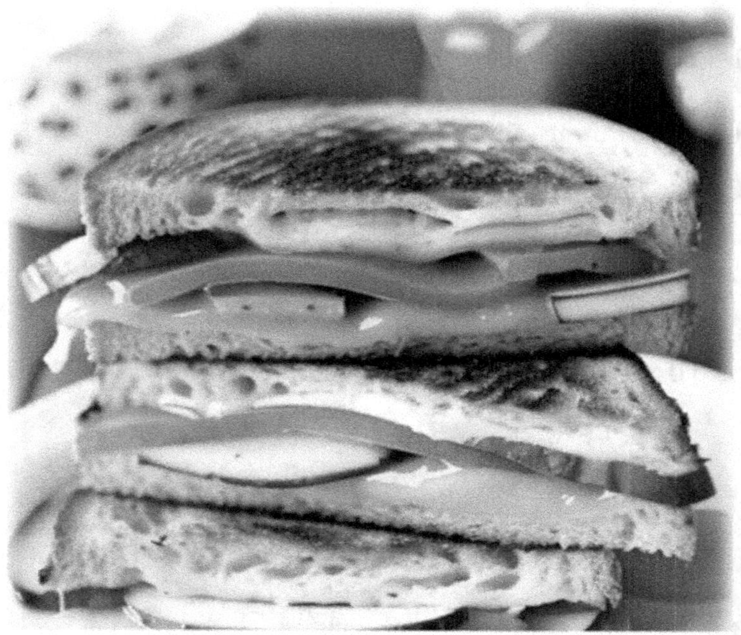

7.Vegetable Fried Brown Rice:

Ingredients:

- 2 cups cooked brown rice

- 2 tablespoons olive oil

- 1/2 cup diced onion

- 1/2 cup diced red bell pepper

- 1/2 cup diced carrots

- 1/2 cup frozen peas

- 2 tablespoons low-sodium soy sauce

- 1/2 teaspoon garlic powder

- Salt and pepper to taste

Instructions:

1. Heat oil in a large skillet over medium heat.

2. Add onion, red pepper, and carrots and cook until softened, about 5 minutes.

3. Add peas, cooked brown rice, soy sauce, and garlic powder. Cook, stirring occasionally, until vegetables are tender, and rice is heated through, about 5 minutes.

4. Taste and season with salt and pepper as desired.

5. Serve warm. Enjoy!

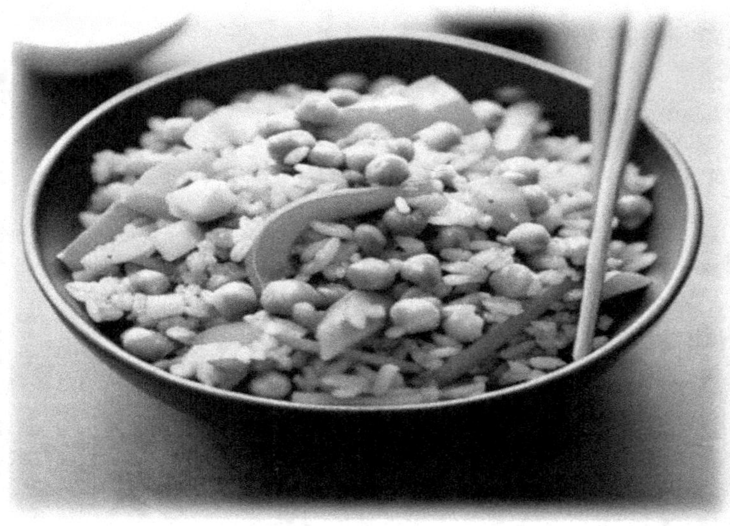

8.Mac and Cheese with Broccoli:

Ingredients:

- ❖ 2 cups macaroni noodles
- ❖ 2-3 tablespoons butter
- ❖ 2 tablespoons all-purpose flour
- ❖ 2 cups milk
- ❖ 1/2 teaspoon salt
- ❖ 1/4 teaspoon pepper
- ❖ 2 cups shredded cheese
- ❖ 2 cups cooked broccoli

Instructions:

1. Preheat oven to 375 degrees F.

2. Cook macaroni according to package instructions.

3. In a medium pot, melt butter over medium heat. Add flour and whisk constantly for 1-2 minutes.

4. Slowly add milk, whisking constantly until mixture is smooth and thickened.

5. Add salt and pepper.

6. Add cheese and stir until melted.

7. Add cooked macaroni noodles and cooked broccoli to the cheese sauce.

8. Grease a 9-inch baking dish. Pour macaroni and cheese mixture into the dish.

9. Bake for 20 minutes until cheese is melted and bubbly.

10. Enjoy!

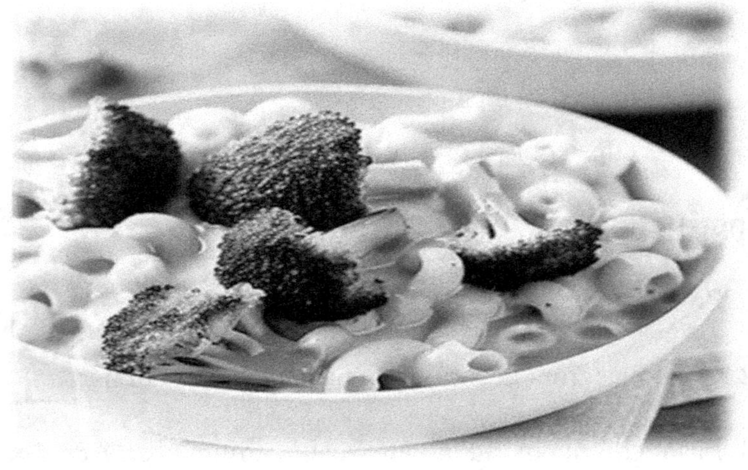

9.Cheesy Baked Zucchini Fritters:

Ingredients:

- 2 cups grated zucchini

- 2 tablespoons olive oil

- 2 tablespoons minced garlic

- 1/2 teaspoon salt

- 1/4 teaspoon freshly ground black pepper

- 1/2 cup grated Parmesan cheese

- 1/2 cup all-purpose flour

- 2 tablespoons chopped fresh parsley

- 2 eggs, lightly beaten

Instructions:

1. Preheat the oven to 375 degrees F.

2. In a large bowl, combine the zucchini, olive oil, garlic, salt, pepper, Parmesan cheese, flour, and parsley.

3. Add the eggs and mix until everything is well combined.

4. Grease a baking sheet with cooking spray.

5. Form the zucchini mixture into small patties and place onto the baking sheet.

6. Bake for 15-20 minutes, or until golden brown and cooked through.

7. Serve warm with a side of your favorite dipping sauce. Enjoy!

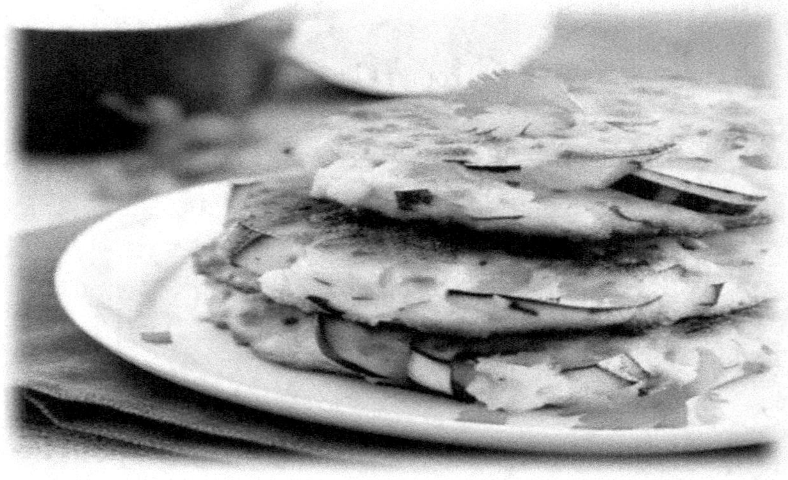

10.Creamy White Bean and Spinach Soup

Ingredients:

- ❖ 2 tablespoons olive oil
- ❖ 1 onion, diced
- ❖ 2 cloves garlic, minced
- ❖ 2 carrots, peeled and diced
- ❖ 1 celery stalk, diced
- ❖ 1 teaspoon dried thyme
- ❖ 2 cans white beans, drained and rinsed
- ❖ 1 cup vegetable broth
- ❖ 2 cups baby spinach leaves
- ❖ Salt and freshly ground black pepper, to taste
- ❖ Freshly chopped parsley, for garnish

Instructions:

1. Heat the olive oil in a large pot over medium heat. Add the onion and garlic and cook for about 3 minutes, until softened.

2. Add the carrots, celery, and thyme and cook for another 3 minutes.

3. Add the white beans and vegetable broth and bring to a boil. Reduce the heat and simmer for about 10 minutes.

4. Add the spinach and cook for another 2 minutes.

5. Season with salt and pepper, to taste.

6. Serve garnished with freshly chopped parsley. Enjoy!

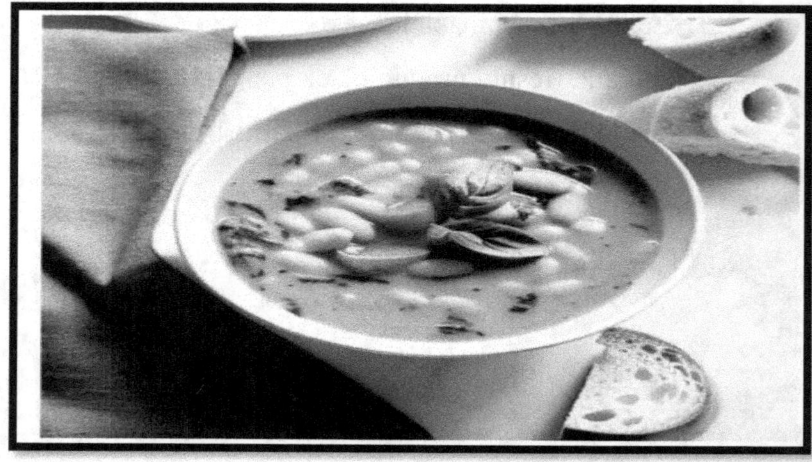

Snacks

This section is filled with nutritionally balanced recipes that provide healthy snack options that are both tasty and fun for kids with cancer.

Our recipes are designed to provide necessary nutrients while also making mealtime enjoyable. Each snack is designed to provide the right amount of energy and nutrients for kids with cancer without adding extra fat or sugar. We also take into account any food allergies or sensitivities that may be present.

We understand that snacks are an important part of a child's diet and can make a difference in their overall wellbeing. That's why we've created this section of recipes that are both healthy and delicious. From energy-boosting smoothies to protein-packed energy bites, this section will help you find the perfect snack for any occasion.

We hope these recipes will make snack time a fun and tasty part of your day. Enjoy!

1.Chocolate Avocado Pudding

Ingredients:

- ❖ 1 ripe avocado
- ❖ 2 tablespoons cocoa powder
- ❖ 2 tablespoons honey
- ❖ 2 tablespoons plain Greek yogurt
- ❖ 1 teaspoon vanilla extract
- ❖ Milk (optional)

Instructions:

1. Cut the avocado in half, remove the pit, and scoop out the flesh into a blender or food processor.

2. Add the cocoa powder, honey, yogurt, and vanilla extract.

3. Blend until smooth and creamy. If needed, add a tablespoon or two of milk to thin out the mixture.

4. Serve chilled in individual bowls or plastic cups. Enjoy!

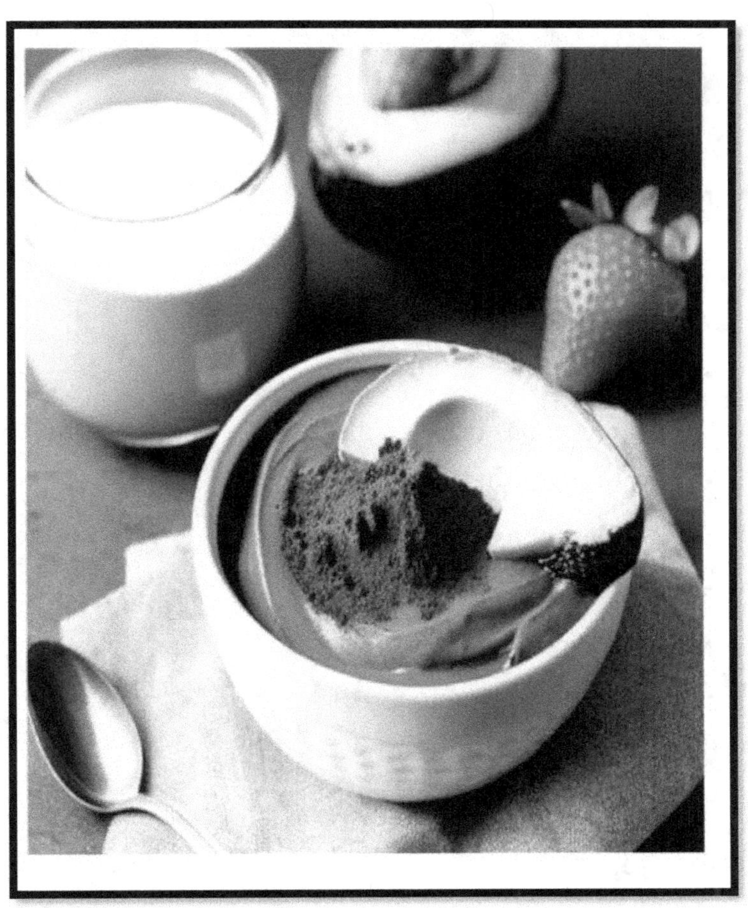

2.Fruity Oatmeal Bites

Ingredients:

- ❖ ½ cup rolled oats
- ❖ ½ cup almond or coconut milk
- ❖ 1 banana
- ❖ 2 tablespoons dried cranberries
- ❖ 2 tablespoons chopped walnuts
- ❖ 2 tablespoons sunflower seeds
- ❖ 2 tablespoons ground flaxseed
- ❖ 2 tablespoons honey
- ❖ 1 teaspoon cinnamon

Instructions:

1. Preheat oven to 350 degrees F.

2. In a medium bowl, mash banana until smooth.

3. Add the oats, milk, cranberries, walnuts, sunflower seeds, flaxseed, honey, and cinnamon. Stir until all ingredients are well combined.

4. Grease a baking sheet with cooking spray.

5. Scoop the mixture onto the baking sheet and form into small bite-sized balls.

6. Bake for 25 minutes, or until edges are golden brown.

7. Serve and enjoy!

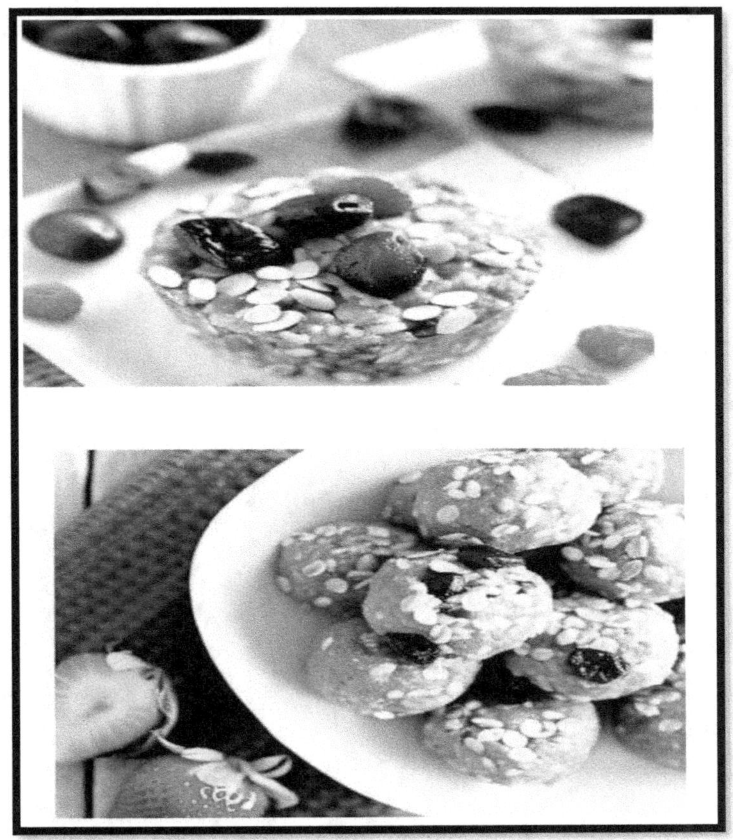

3.Peanut Butter & Apple Roll-Ups

Ingredients:

- ❖ 1 large apple, cored and thinly sliced
- ❖ 2 tablespoons natural peanut butter
- ❖ 2 tablespoons honey
- ❖ 1 tablespoon ground flaxseed
- ❖ Dash of cinnamon

Instructions:

1. Spread the peanut butter on each apple slice.

2. Drizzle honey over the peanut butter.

3. Sprinkle flaxseed and cinnamon on top.

4. Roll the apple slices and secure with a toothpick.

5. Serve and enjoy!

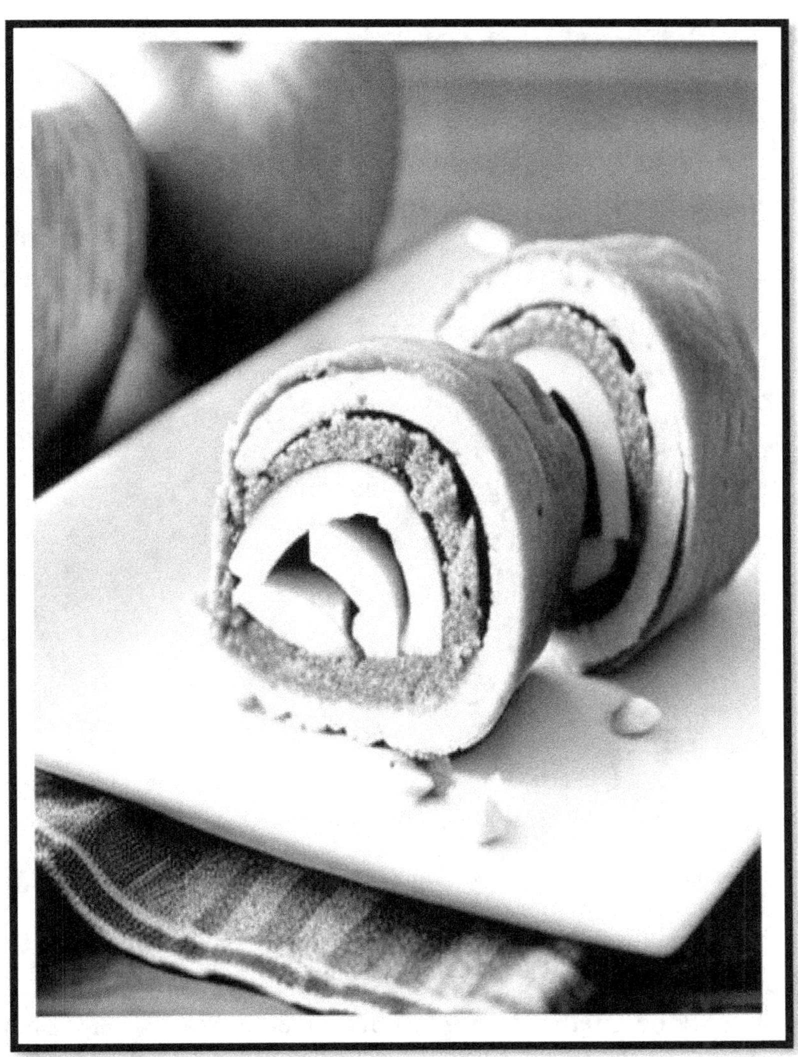

4.Chocolate Oatmeal Bites

Ingredients:

- 1 cup rolled oats
- 1/4 cup almond butter
- 1/4 cup honey
- 3 tablespoons cocoa powder
- 1/4 teaspoon ground cinnamon
- 1/4 teaspoon vanilla extract
- 1/4 cup mini chocolate chips

Instructions:

1. In a medium bowl, mix together the oats, almond butter, honey, cocoa powder, cinnamon, and vanilla extract.

2. Stir in the mini chocolate chips.

3. Roll the mixture into small bite-sized balls and place on a baking sheet lined with parchment paper.

4. Place the baking sheet in the refrigerator for at least 1 hour.

5. Enjoy your delicious Chocolate Oatmeal Bites!

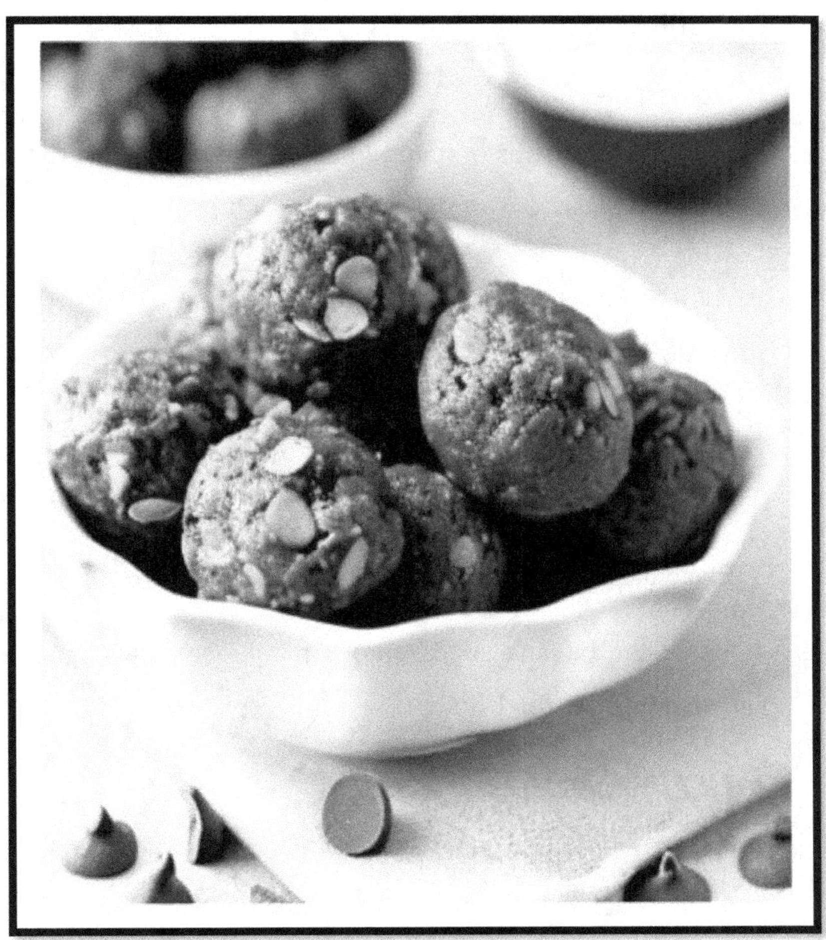

5.Chocolate Banana Bites

Ingredients:

- ❖ 1 large banana
- ❖ 2 tablespoons of natural peanut butter
- ❖ 2 tablespoons of dark chocolate chips

Instructions:

1. Slice the banana into ½-inch thick slices.

2. Spread a small amount of peanut butter onto each slice.

3. Place dark chocolate chips onto the peanut butter.

4. Place the banana slices onto a parchment-lined baking sheet and freeze for 1 hour.

5. Serve and enjoy!

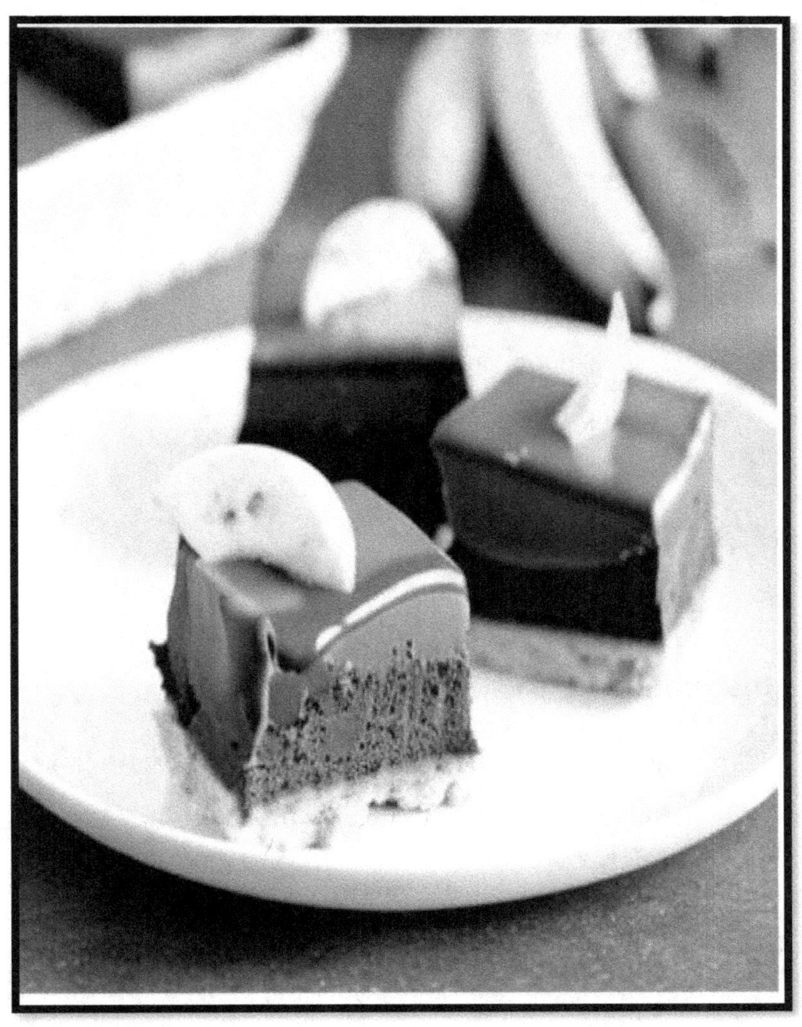

6.Fruity Yogurt Bites

Ingredients:

- ❖ 2 cups plain Greek yogurt
- ❖ 2 tablespoons honey
- ❖ 1/2 teaspoon vanilla extract
- ❖ 1/2 cup fresh blueberries
- ❖ 1/2 cup fresh raspberries
- ❖ 1/4 cup chopped almonds

Instructions:

1. In a medium bowl, mix together the Greek yogurt, honey and vanilla extract until completely combined.

2. Gently fold in the blueberries, raspberries and almonds.

3. Spoon the mixture into a lined muffin tin, filling each cup about 3/4 full.

4. Freeze the muffin tin for at least 4 hours or overnight.

5. When ready to serve, remove the Fruity Yogurt Bites from the muffin tin and enjoy!

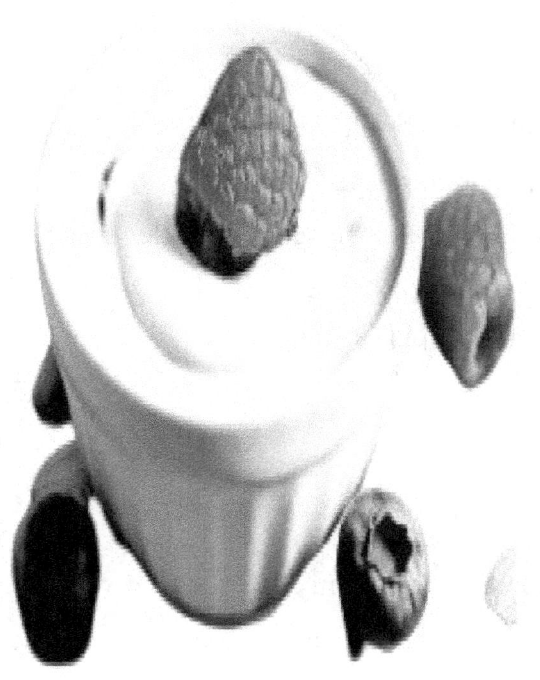

7.Healthy Fruit and Nut Bites

Ingredients:

- ❖ 1/2 cup of walnuts, chopped
- ❖ 1/2 cup of almonds, chopped
- ❖ 1/4 cup of dried cranberries
- ❖ 1/4 cup of dried blueberries
- ❖ 1/4 cup of raisins
- ❖ 1/4 cup of unsweetened shredded coconut
- ❖ 2 tablespoons of hemp seeds
- ❖ 1/4 cup of almond butter

Instructions:

1. In a medium bowl, mix together the walnuts, almonds, cranberries, blueberries, raisins, and shredded coconut.

2. Add the hemp seeds and almond butter and mix until all ingredients are well combined.

3. Using your hands, shape the mixture into bite-sized balls.

4. Place the balls on a parchment-lined baking sheet and chill in the refrigerator for at least 20 minutes.

5. Enjoy your healthy fruit and nut bites!

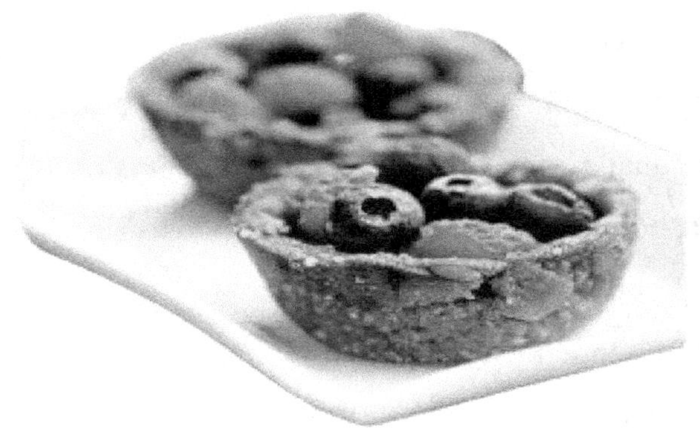

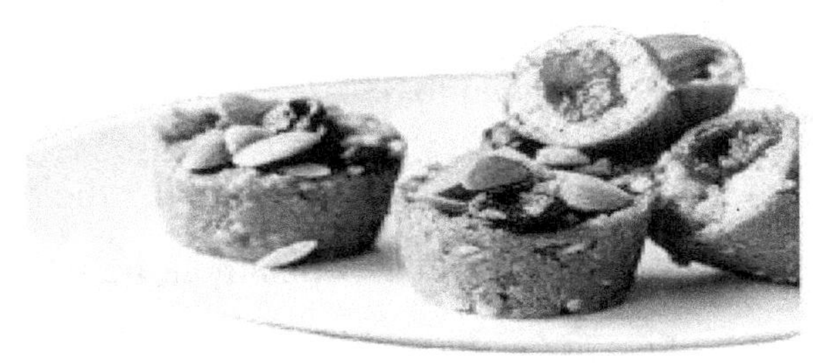

8.Healthy Banana Oat Bars

Ingredients:

- ❖ 2 cups rolled oats
- ❖ 1/4 cup melted coconut oil
- ❖ 2 ripe bananas, mashed
- ❖ 1/4 teaspoon ground cinnamon
- ❖ 1/4 cup honey
- ❖ 1/4 cup chopped walnuts
- ❖ 1/4 cup dried cranberries

Instructions:

1. Preheat oven to 350°F.

2. In a medium bowl, mix together the oats, melted coconut oil, mashed bananas, cinnamon, honey, walnuts, and dried cranberries.

3. Grease an 8x8 baking pan with coconut oil.

4. Pour the oat mixture into the greased pan and spread evenly.

5. Bake in preheated oven for 20-25 minutes until lightly golden brown.

6. Allow to cool completely before cutting into bars.

Enjoy!

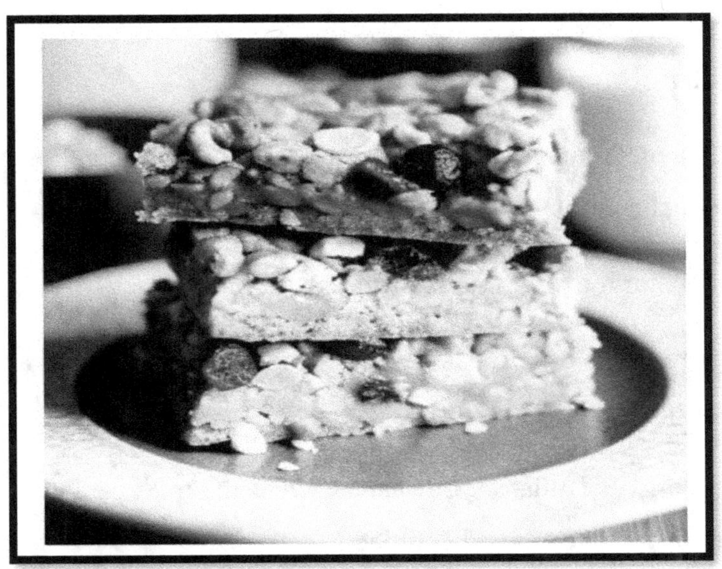

9.No-Bake Chocolate Peanut Butter Granola Bars

Ingredients:

- ❖ 2 cups rolled oats
- ❖ 1/2 cup natural peanut butter
- ❖ 1/3 cup honey
- ❖ 1/2 cup dark chocolate chips
- ❖ 1/4 cup ground flaxseed
- ❖ 1/4 cup unsweetened coconut flakes (optional)
- ❖ 1 teaspoon vanilla extract

Instructions:

1. In a medium bowl, combine the oats, peanut butter, honey, chocolate chips, flaxseed, and coconut flakes (if using).

2. Mix until everything is evenly combined.

3. Line an 8x8 inch baking dish with parchment paper and pour the mixture into the pan.

4. Using a spatula or your hands, press the mixture into the pan until it is even and compact.

5. Place the pan in the refrigerator and let it chill for at least 1 hour.

6. Remove the pan from the refrigerator and cut into bars.

7. Store in an airtight container in the refrigerator for up to 1 week. Enjoy!

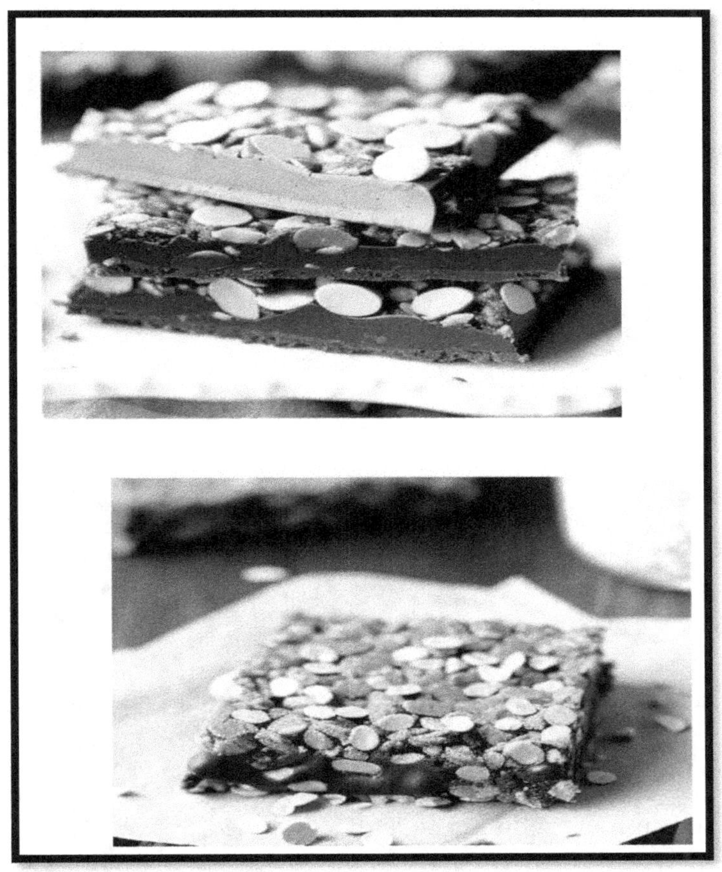

10.Fruit and Nut Bites

Ingredients:

• 2 tablespoons of honey

• 1/2 teaspoon of cinnamon

• 2 tablespoons of peanut butter

• 2 tablespoons of ground flaxseed

• 1/4 cup of chopped nuts (almonds, walnuts, etc.)

• 1/4 cup of raisins

• 1/4 cup of dried cranberries

Instructions:

1. In a small bowl, combine honey, cinnamon, peanut butter and flaxseed.

2. Stir until everything is evenly combined.

3. Add in the nuts, raisins and cranberries and mix everything together.

4. Using a spoon or a small ice cream scoop, scoop out small mounds of the mixture onto a baking sheet lined with parchment paper.

5. Place the baking sheet into the refrigerator and chill for at least 1 hour.

6. Serve and enjoy!

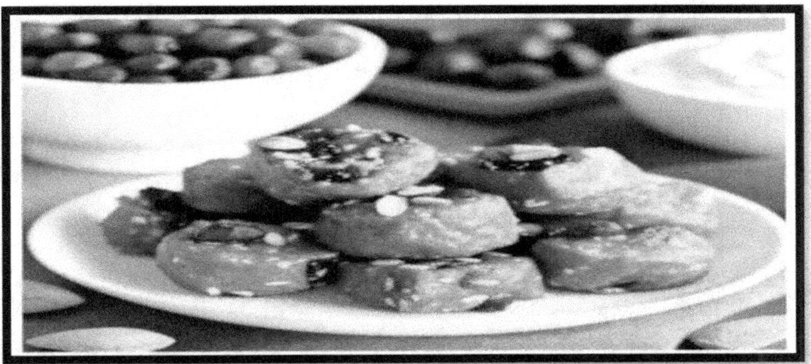

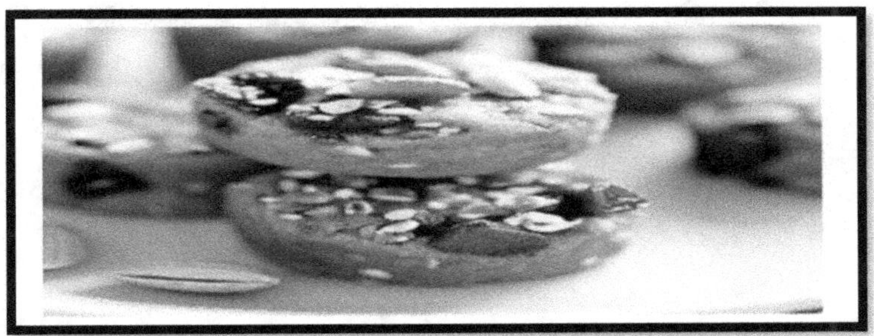

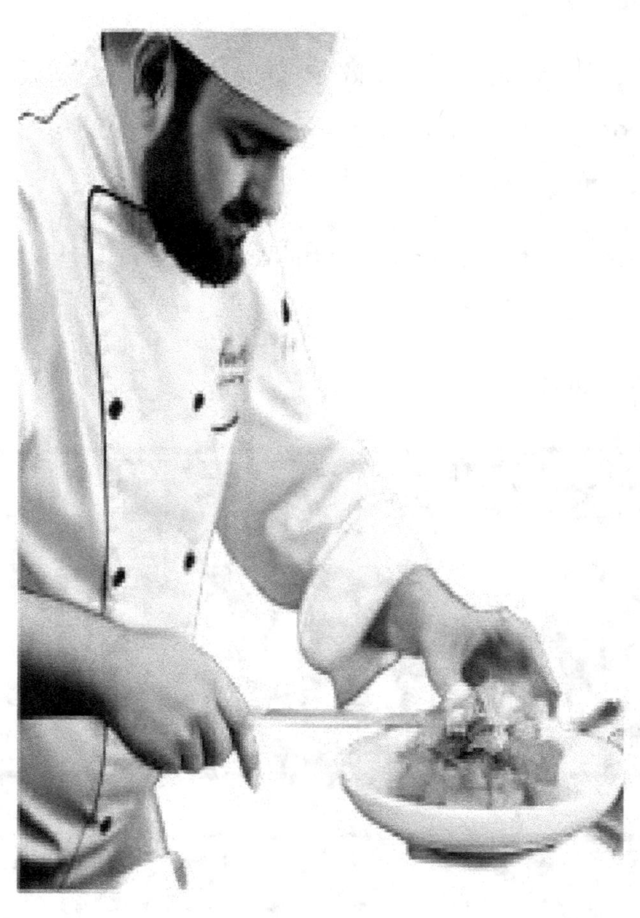

Dinner

Eating a well-balanced diet is important for all children, but especially so for kids with cancer. Eating the right foods can help improve their overall health and well-being, as well as support their body in fighting the cancer.

This dinner recipes guide is designed to provide a variety of easy and nutritious dinner ideas for kids with cancer. It includes delicious, cancer-fighting ingredients like fruits and vegetables, lean proteins, healthy fats, and whole grains. All of the recipes are also free of added sugars and processed foods, both of which can have a negative effect on a child's health.

The recipes are intended to be simple, easy to make, and enjoyable for kids of all ages. In addition, each recipe includes nutrition facts to help make it easier for parents to track the nutritional value of their child's meals.

We hope that these recipes will help make dinner time a fun, nutritious, and cancer-fighting experience for your child. Bon Appétit!

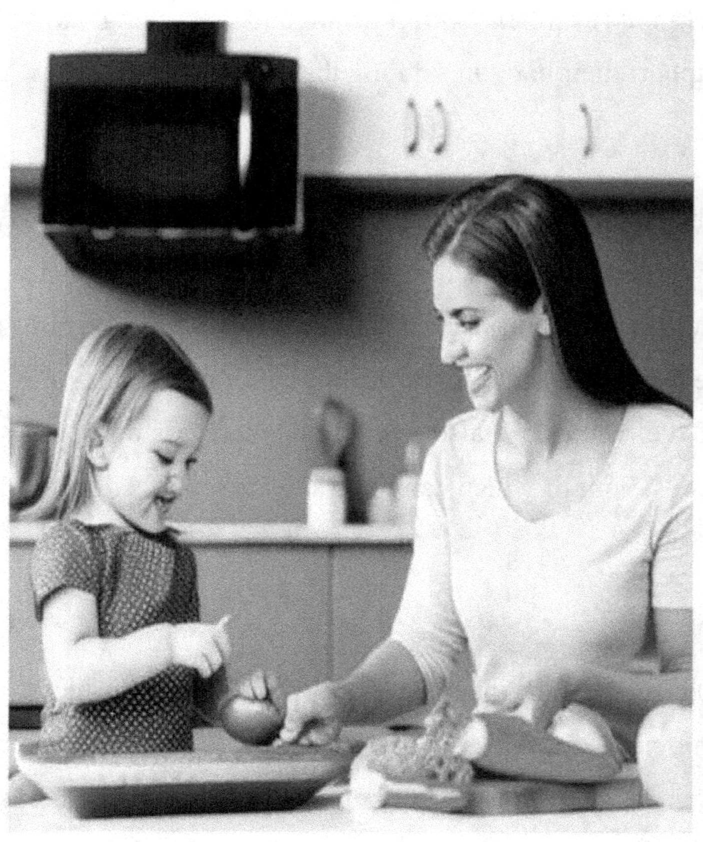

1.Veggie Quinoa Burrito Bowls

Ingredients:

- ❖ 1 tablespoon olive oil
- ❖ 1 cup uncooked quinoa
- ❖ 2 cups vegetable broth
- ❖ 1 red bell pepper, diced
- ❖ 1 green bell pepper, diced
- ❖ 1 onion, diced
- ❖ 1 can black beans, drained and rinsed
- ❖ 1 can corn, drained
- ❖ 1 teaspoon cumin
- ❖ 1 teaspoon chili powder
- ❖ 1 teaspoon garlic powder
- ❖ Salt and pepper, to taste
- ❖ 1/2 cup shredded cheese
- ❖ 1/2 cup salsa
- ❖ 1/4 cup chopped cilantro
- ❖ 1 avocado, diced

Instructions:

1. Heat the olive oil in a large pot over medium heat.

2. Add the quinoa and stir to coat in the oil.

3. Pour in the vegetable broth and bring to a boil.

4. Reduce the heat to low and simmer, covered, for 15 minutes.

5. Meanwhile, in a large skillet, heat the remaining olive oil over medium-high heat.

6. Add the bell peppers, onion, black beans, corn, cumin, chili powder, garlic powder, salt, and pepper.

7. Cook, stirring occasionally, until the vegetables are tender, about 8 minutes.

8. When the quinoa is done, fluff with a fork and stir in the vegetable mixture.

9. Divide the quinoa between 4 bowls and top with cheese, salsa, cilantro, and avocado.

10. Serve warm. Enjoy!

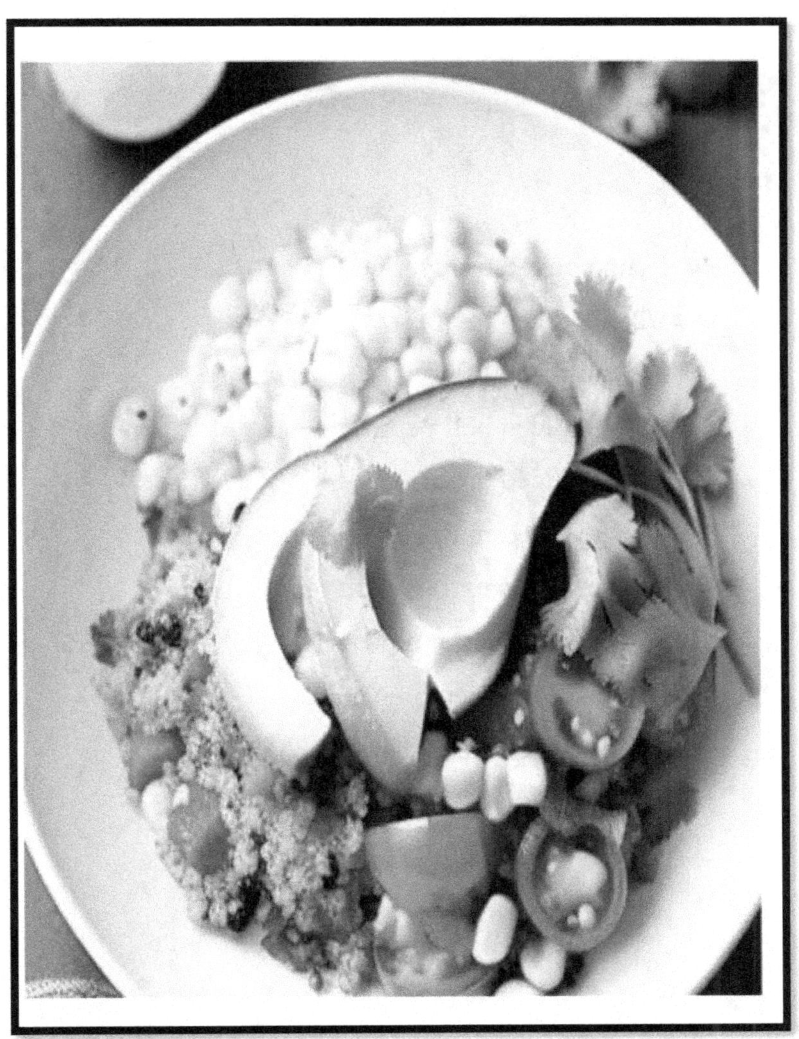

2.Veggie Brown Rice Bowl

Ingredients:

- ❖ 1 cup cooked brown rice
- ❖ 1/2 cup diced carrots
- ❖ 1/2 cup diced celery
- ❖ 1/2 cup diced bell pepper
- ❖ 1/2 cup diced onion
- ❖ 1/2 cup diced mushrooms
- ❖ 2 tablespoons extra-virgin olive oil
- ❖ 1/2 teaspoon garlic powder
- ❖ 1/2 teaspoon dried oregano
- ❖ 1/4 teaspoon sea salt

Instructions:

1. Heat olive oil in a large skillet over medium heat.

2. Add the diced carrots, celery, bell pepper, onion, and mushrooms.

3. Sauté the vegetables for 5 minutes, stirring occasionally.

4. Add the garlic powder, oregano, and sea salt.

5. Sauté for an additional 5 minutes.

6. Serve the vegetables over the cooked brown rice. Enjoy!

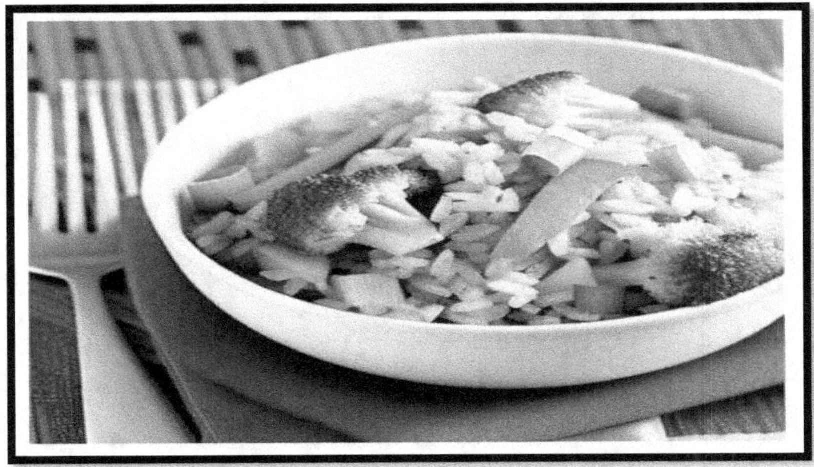

3.Vegetable and Lentil Stew

Ingredients:

- ❖ 1 cup dried green lentils, rinsed
- ❖ 1 onion, diced
- ❖ 3 cloves garlic, minced
- ❖ 1 cup diced carrots
- ❖ 1 cup diced celery
- ❖ 1 teaspoon dried oregano
- ❖ 1 teaspoon dried thyme
- ❖ 1 bay leaf
- ❖ 2 tablespoons tomato paste
- ❖ 4 cups vegetable broth
- ❖ 1/2 teaspoon salt
- ❖ 1/4 teaspoon black pepper
- ❖ 1/2 cup frozen green peas

Instructions:

1. Heat a large soup pot over medium heat. Add the onion and garlic and sauté for 5 minutes, until the onion is softened.

2. Add the carrots, celery, oregano, thyme, and bay leaf and sauté for an additional 5 minutes.

3. Stir in the tomato paste and cook for 1 minute.

4. Add the lentils, vegetable broth, salt, and pepper. Bring the mixture to a boil, then reduce the heat to low and simmer for 30 minutes, uncovered, stirring occasionally.

5. Add the frozen peas and cook for an additional 5 minutes.

6. Serve the stew with a side of cooked grains, such as quinoa or brown rice. Enjoy!

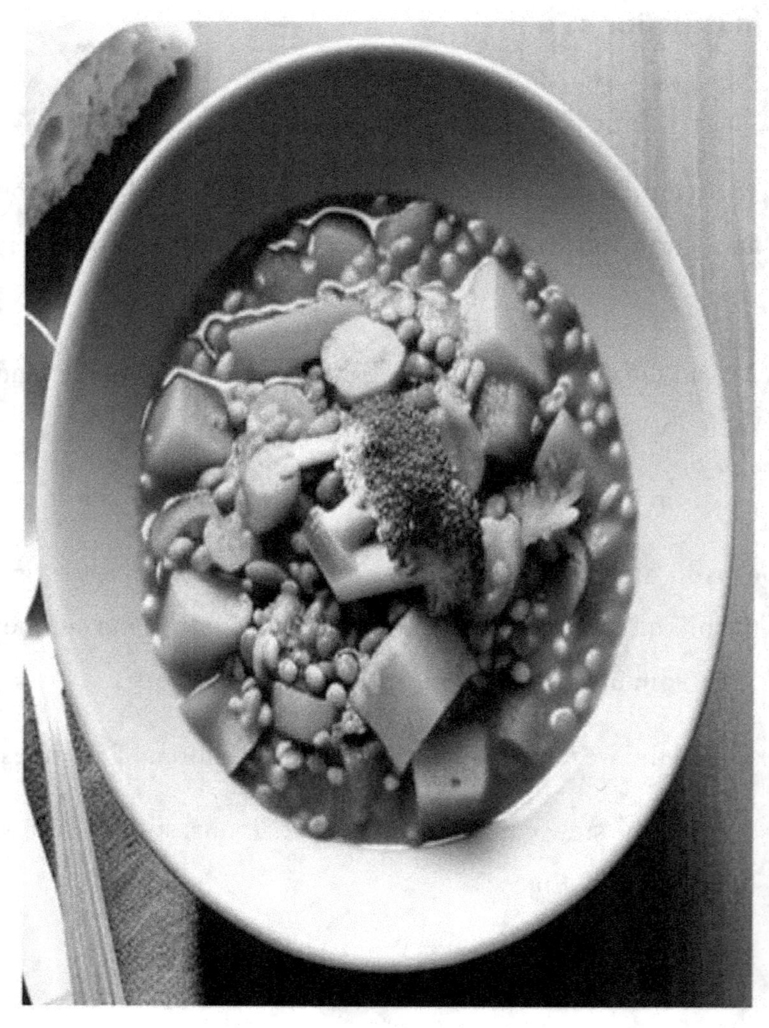

4.Lentil and Sweet Potato Curry

Ingredients:

- ❖ 1 cup dried lentils, rinsed and drained
- ❖ 2 tablespoons olive oil
- ❖ 1 medium onion, diced
- ❖ 2 cloves garlic, minced
- ❖ 1 teaspoon ground cumin
- ❖ 1 teaspoon ground coriander
- ❖ 1/2 teaspoon ground turmeric
- ❖ 1/4 teaspoon ground cinnamon
- ❖ 1/4 teaspoon ground cardamom
- ❖ 1/4 teaspoon ground ginger
- ❖ 1/2 teaspoon salt
- ❖ 2 cups vegetable broth
- ❖ 2 cups diced sweet potatoes
- ❖ 1 cup diced tomatoes
- ❖ 1/2 cup frozen green peas
- ❖ 2 tablespoons chopped fresh cilantro

Instructions:

1. Heat the olive oil in a large Dutch oven or stockpot over medium heat. Add the onion and garlic and cook, stirring occasionally, until softened, about 5 minutes.

2. Stir in the cumin, coriander, turmeric, cinnamon, cardamom, ginger, and salt and cook for 1 minute.

3. Add the lentils, broth, sweet potatoes, and tomatoes and bring to a boil. Reduce the heat to low, cover, and simmer for 20 minutes, or until the lentils and sweet potatoes are tender.

4. Stir in the peas and cilantro, cover, and simmer for 5 minutes more.

5. Serve over cooked rice or quinoa, if desired. Enjoy!

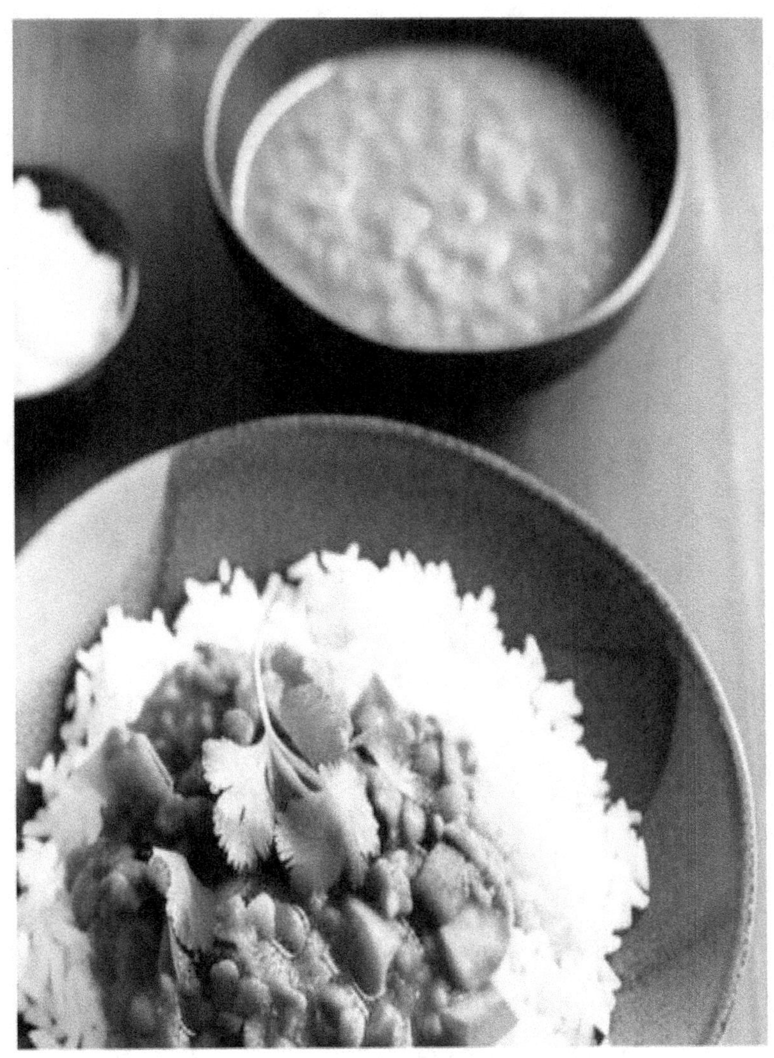

5.Lentil and Sweet Potato Stew

Ingredients:

- ❖ 1 tablespoon olive oil
- ❖ 1 medium onion, diced
- ❖ 2 cloves garlic, minced
- ❖ 1 teaspoon dried thyme
- ❖ 1 teaspoon smoked paprika
- ❖ 1/2 teaspoon ground cumin
- ❖ 1/4 teaspoon ground coriander
- ❖ 3 cups vegetable broth
- ❖ 2 cups cooked lentils
- ❖ 2 medium sweet potatoes, peeled and diced
- ❖ 2 carrots, peeled and diced
- ❖ 1 red bell pepper, diced
- ❖ 1 cup diced zucchini
- ❖ 1/4 cup chopped fresh parsley

Instructions:

1. Heat the oil in a large pot over medium heat. Add the onion and cook until softened, about 5 minutes.

2. Add the garlic, thyme, paprika, cumin, and coriander and cook for 1 minute, stirring continuously.

3. Add the vegetable broth, lentils, sweet potatoes, carrots, bell pepper, and zucchini and bring to a boil. Reduce the heat to low and simmer until the vegetables are tender, about 20 minutes.

4. Add the parsley and cook for an additional 5 minutes. Serve warm.

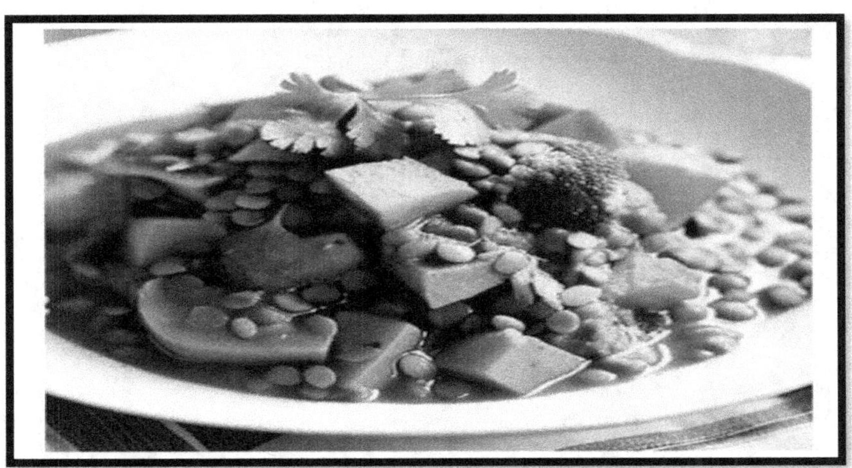

6.Lentil Sloppy Joes

Ingredients:

- ❖ 1 tablespoon olive oil
- ❖ 1 onion, diced
- ❖ 2 cloves garlic, minced
- ❖ 1 cup dried lentils, rinsed
- ❖ 2 cups vegetable broth
- ❖ 1 teaspoon Italian seasoning
- ❖ 1 tablespoon Worcestershire sauce
- ❖ 1 tablespoon tomato paste
- ❖ 1/2 teaspoon brown sugar
- ❖ 1/2 teaspoon smoked paprika
- ❖ 1/4 teaspoon salt
- ❖ 1/4 teaspoon black pepper
- ❖ 1/4 cup water
- ❖ 2 tablespoons apple cider vinegar
- ❖ 1 tablespoon Dijon mustard
- ❖ 4 whole wheat hamburger buns

Instructions:

1. Heat the olive oil in a large skillet over medium heat. Add the onion and garlic and cook until softened, about 5 minutes.

2. Add the lentils and vegetable broth and bring to a simmer. Cover and cook for 20 minutes, stirring occasionally, until the lentils are tender.

3. Add the Italian seasoning, Worcestershire sauce, tomato paste, brown sugar, smoked paprika, salt, and pepper and stir to combine.

4. Add the water, vinegar, and mustard and stir to combine. Simmer for 10 minutes, stirring occasionally.

5. Serve the lentil mixture on whole wheat hamburger buns. Enjoy!

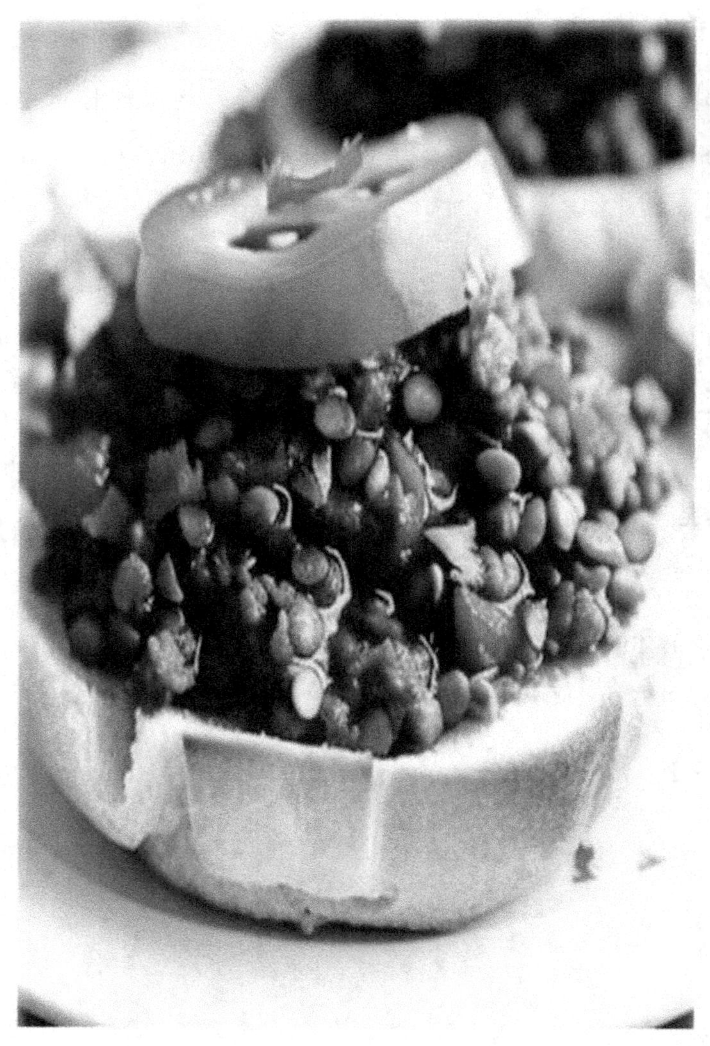

7. Whole Grain Macaroni and Cheese with Broccoli

Ingredients:

- ❖ 2 cups of whole grain elbow macaroni
- ❖ 2 cups of broccoli florets
- ❖ 2 tablespoons of butter
- ❖ 2 tablespoons of all-purpose flour
- ❖ 2 cups of milk
- ❖ 2 cups of shredded cheddar cheese
- ❖ 1 teaspoon of garlic powder
- ❖ Salt and pepper to taste

Directions:

1. Preheat oven to 375°F.

2. Bring a large pot of salted water to a boil. Add the macaroni and cook for 8 minutes. Add the broccoli and cook for an additional 3 minutes. Drain the macaroni and broccoli and set aside.

3. In a large pot, melt the butter over medium heat. Whisk in the flour and cook for 1 minute. Slowly whisk in the milk, stirring constantly until the mixture is smooth. Increase the heat to medium-high and bring the mixture to a simmer.

4. Reduce the heat to low and add the cheese, garlic powder, salt and pepper, stirring until the cheese is melted. Add the macaroni and broccoli and stir until everything is evenly coated.

5. Transfer the mixture to a 9x13 inch baking dish. Bake for 25 minutes, or until the top is golden brown. Serve warm.

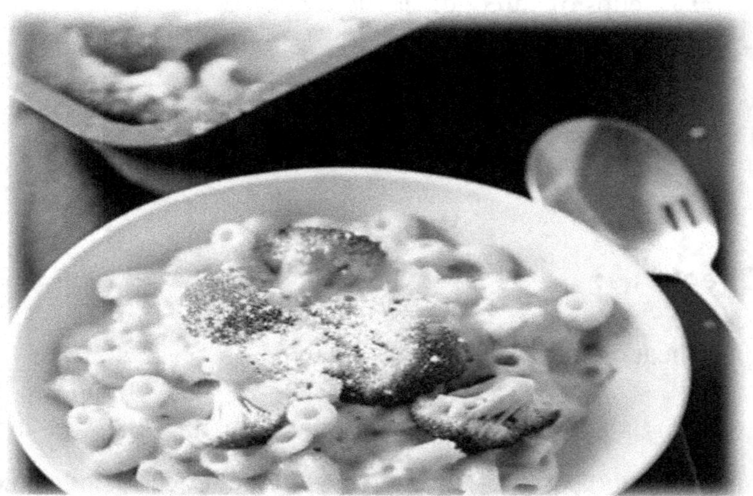

8.Turkey and Whole Grain Pilaf

Ingredients:

- ❖ 2 tablespoons olive oil
- ❖ 1 medium onion, diced
- ❖ 1 clove garlic, minced
- ❖ 1 cup uncooked brown rice
- ❖ 2 cups low-sodium chicken broth
- ❖ 1/2 cup uncooked quinoa
- ❖ 1/4 teaspoon ground turmeric
- ❖ 1/4 teaspoon ground cumin
- ❖ 1/4 teaspoon ground coriander
- ❖ 1/4 teaspoon ground cinnamon
- ❖ 1/2 teaspoon sea salt
- ❖ 1/2 pound ground turkey
- ❖ 1 cup frozen peas
- ❖ 1/4 cup chopped fresh parsley

Instructions:

1. Heat the olive oil in a large saucepan over medium-high heat. Add the onion and garlic, and cook, stirring frequently, for about 5 minutes, or until the onion is softened and lightly browned.

2. Add the brown rice, chicken broth, quinoa, turmeric, cumin, coriander, cinnamon, and salt. Bring to a boil, then reduce the heat to low, cover, and simmer for 30 minutes, or until the rice and quinoa are cooked through.

3. While the rice is cooking, heat a separate large skillet over medium-high heat. Add the ground turkey and cook, stirring occasionally, until the turkey is cooked through, about 10 minutes.

4. Once the turkey is cooked through, add it to the cooked rice and quinoa along with the frozen peas. Cover the pan and cook for an additional 5 minutes, or until the peas are heated through.

5. Serve the pilaf warm, garnished with the fresh parsley. Enjoy!

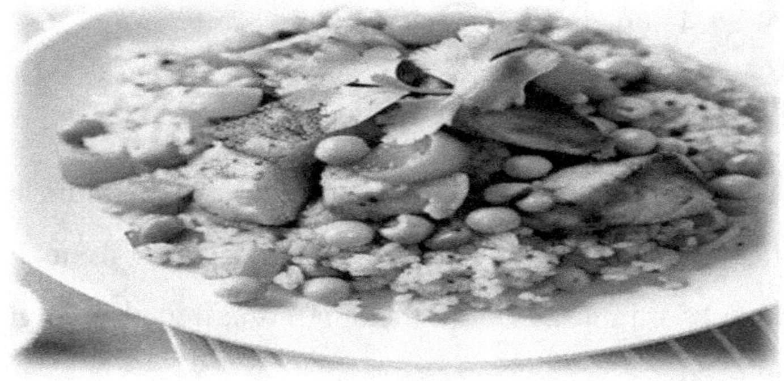

9.Cinnamon Apple Quinoa

Ingredients :

- ❖ 1 cup quinoa
- ❖ 2 cups water
- ❖ 2 tablespoons olive oil
- ❖ 1/2 teaspoon ground cinnamon
- ❖ 2 apples, diced
- ❖ 1/4 cup raisins
- ❖ 2 tablespoons honey
- ❖ 1/4 teaspoon salt

Instructions:

1. In a medium saucepan, bring the quinoa and water to a boil over medium-high heat. Reduce heat to low, cover, and simmer for 15 minutes or until the water is absorbed.

2. Heat the olive oil in a large skillet over medium heat. Add the cinnamon, diced apples, and raisins. Cook, stirring occasionally, until the apples are softened, about 5 minutes.

3. Add the cooked quinoa, honey, and salt to the skillet. Cook, stirring occasionally, until heated through, about 5 minutes.

4. Serve the quinoa warm. Enjoy!

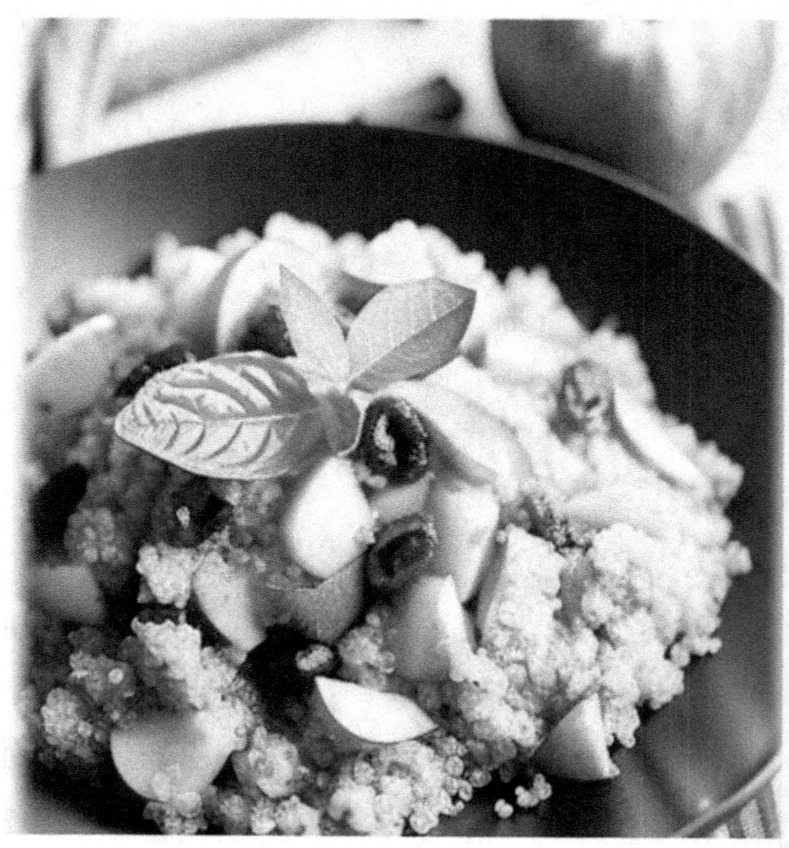

10.Vegetable and Bean Soup:

Ingredients:

- ❖ 2 tablespoons olive oil
- ❖ 1 onion, diced
- ❖ 2 carrots, sliced
- ❖ 2 celery stalks, diced
- ❖ 2 cloves garlic, minced
- ❖ 1 teaspoon dried oregano
- ❖ 1 teaspoon dried basil
- ❖ 4 cups vegetable broth
- ❖ 1 can (14.5 ounces) diced tomatoes
- ❖ 1 can (15 ounces) cannellini beans, drained and rinsed
- ❖ 1 cup frozen corn
- ❖ Salt and pepper, to taste

Instructions:

1. Heat the olive oil in a large pot over medium heat.

2. Add the onion, carrots, and celery and cook until softened, about 5 minutes.

3. Add the garlic, oregano, and basil and cook for 1 minute.

4. Add the vegetable broth, tomatoes, beans, and corn and bring to a simmer.

5. Simmer for 10 minutes, or until the vegetables are tender.

6. Season with salt and pepper, to taste.

7. Serve warm. Enjoy!

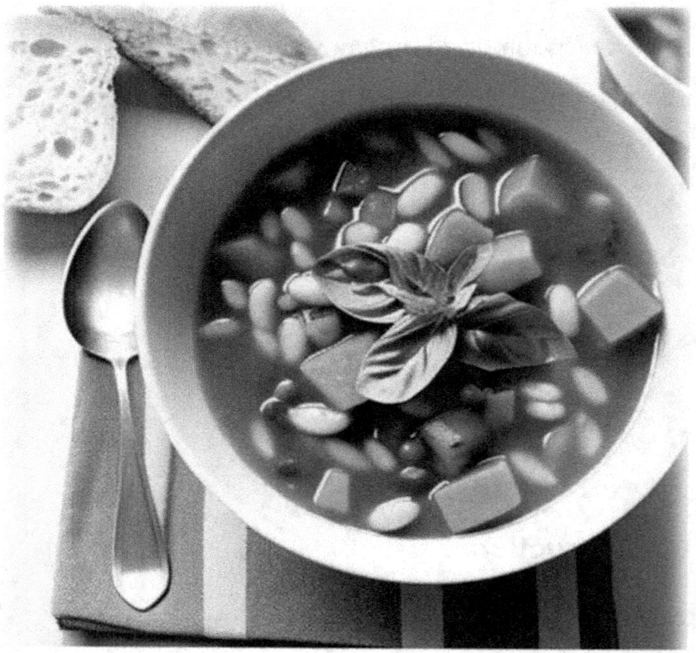

Desserts

We know that having to follow a special diet can be hard, but we're here to show you that it doesn't mean you have to miss out on your favorite sweet treats. We've created delicious and nutritious recipes for cancer-fighting desserts that taste just as good as the real thing. From cakes and cookies to smoothies and ice cream, you'll find plenty of options to satisfy your sweet tooth. Our recipes are designed to be easy to make and use healthy, cancer-fighting ingredients, allowing you to enjoy your favorite desserts without worrying about their impact on your health. So, grab your apron and let's get baking!

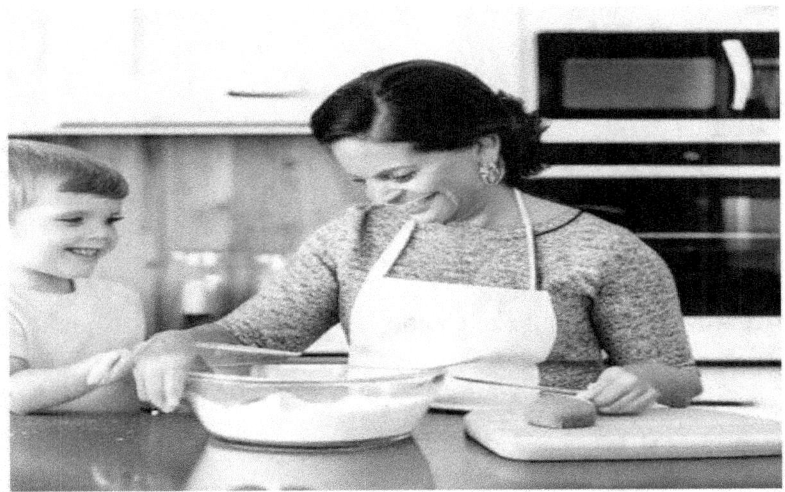

1.No-Bake Chocolate Coconut Cookies

Ingredients:

- ❖ 1/4 cup coconut oil
- ❖ 3/4 cup cocoa powder
- ❖ 1/4 cup maple syrup
- ❖ 1/4 cup unsweetened coconut flakes

Instructions:

1. In a medium bowl, combine the coconut oil, cocoa powder and maple syrup. Stir together until completely mixed together.

2. Add the coconut flakes and stir until evenly distributed.

3. Scoop out tablespoon sized portions of the mixture and roll into balls.

4. Place on a parchment lined baking sheet and press down lightly with your fingertips.

5. Place baking sheet in the freezer for 1 hour.

6. Store in an airtight container in the refrigerator for up to 1 week. Enjoy!

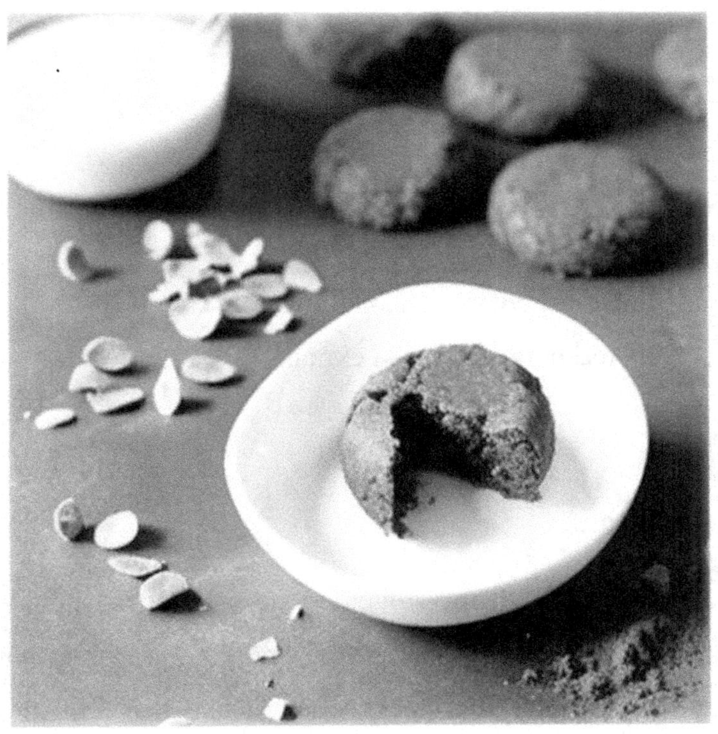

2.No-Bake Chocolate Peanut Butter Bars

Ingredients:

- ❖ 2 cups of gluten-free oats
- ❖ 2 tablespoons of cocoa powder
- ❖ 2 tablespoons of honey
- ❖ 4 tablespoons of peanut butter
- ❖ 2 tablespoons of coconut oil
- ❖ ½ teaspoon of vanilla extract

Instructions:

1. In a large bowl, mix together the oats, cocoa powder, honey, peanut butter, coconut oil, and vanilla extract until they are well combined.

2. Line a 9x13 inch pan with parchment paper and pour the oat mixture into the pan.

3. Press the mixture into the pan firmly and evenly.

4. Place the pan in the freezer and let it set for 1 hour.

5. After an hour, remove the pan from the freezer and cut the oat mixture into bars.

6. Enjoy!

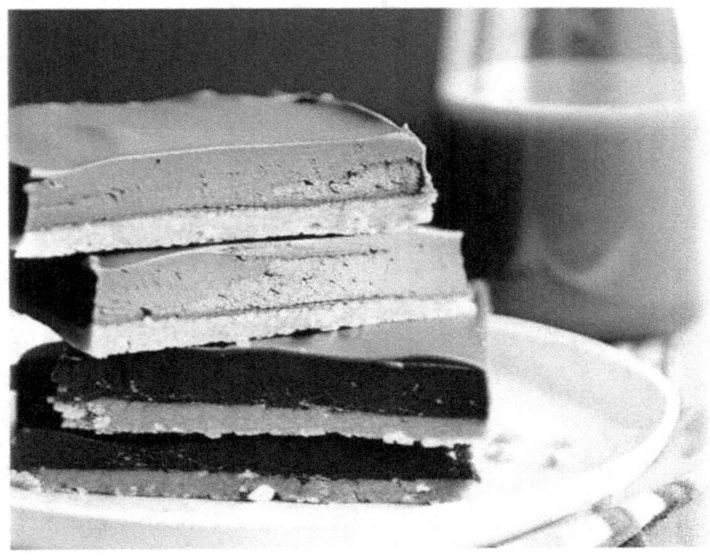

3.Mixed Berry Mousse

Ingredients:

- ❖ 1 cup frozen mixed berries
- ❖ 1/4 cup unsweetened applesauce
- ❖ 1 teaspoon honey
- ❖ 1 teaspoon vanilla extract
- ❖ 1/4 teaspoon ground cinnamon

Instructions:

1. Place the frozen berries in a medium saucepan over medium heat.

2. Cook, stirring occasionally, until the berries are soft and beginning to break down, about 5 minutes.

3. Remove the saucepan from the heat and add the applesauce, honey, vanilla extract, and ground cinnamon. Stir until evenly combined.

4. Transfer the mixture to a blender and blend until smooth.

5. Divide the mousse into individual serving dishes and chill
in the refrigerator for at least 1 hour.

6. Serve chilled and enjoy!

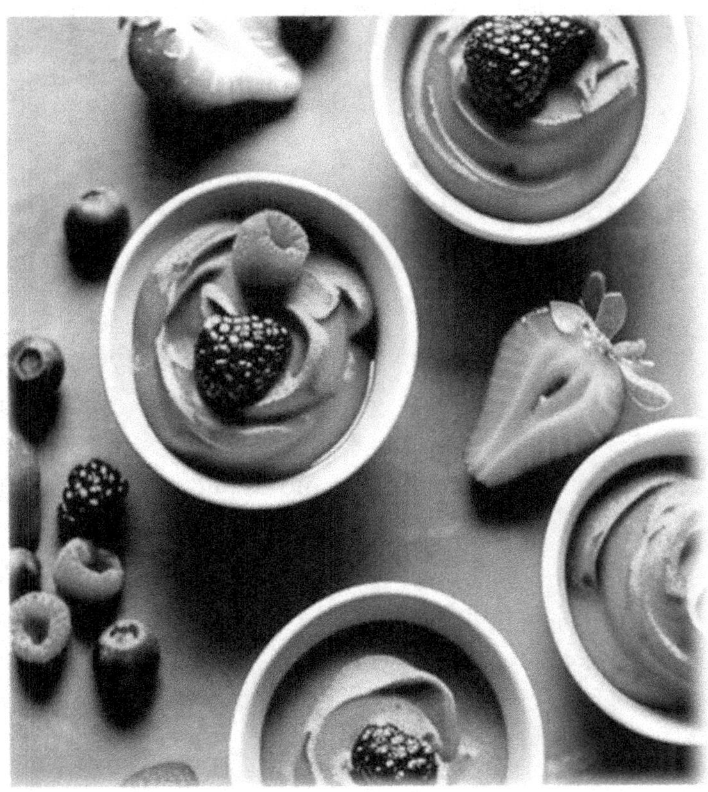

4.Mixed Berry Yogurt Popsicles

Ingredients:

- ❖ 1 cup plain, unsweetened yogurt.
- ❖ 1/4 cup mixed berries (such as raspberries, blueberries, blackberries, and/or strawberries)
- ❖ 2 tablespoons honey

Instructions:

1. In a blender, combine the yogurt, mixed berries, and honey until smooth.

2. Pour the mixture into popsicle molds and freeze for at least 4 hours.

3. To remove the popsicles from the molds, run the outside of the molds under warm water and gently pull the popsicles out.

4. Enjoy!

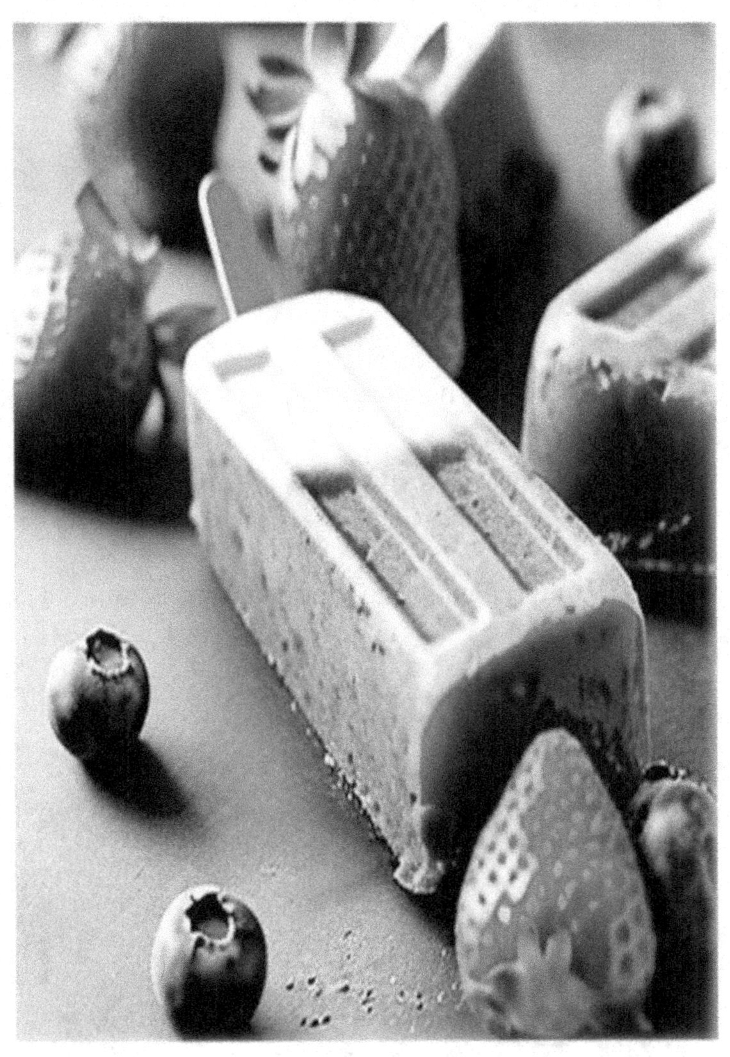

5.Chocolate Banana Soft Serve

Ingredients:

- ❖ 2 ripe bananas
- ❖ 2 tablespoons cocoa powder
- ❖ 1 tablespoon honey

Instructions:

1. Peel and slice the bananas, then place them in a food processor or blender.

2. Add the cocoa powder and honey to the food processor.

3. Blend the ingredients until the mixture is smooth and creamy.

4. Serve the mixture in a bowl or cup and enjoy!

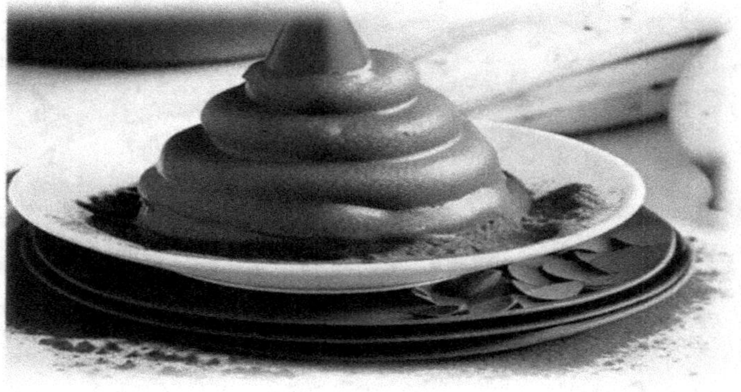

6.Chocolate Coconut Chia Seed Pudding

Ingredients:

- 1/4 cup chia seeds
- 2 cups canned coconut milk
- 2 tablespoons cocoa powder
- 2 tablespoons honey
- 1 teaspoon vanilla extract
- 2 tablespoons shredded coconut
- 1/4 teaspoon ground cinnamon (optional)

Instructions:

1. In a medium bowl, whisk together the chia seeds, coconut milk, cocoa powder, honey, and vanilla extract.

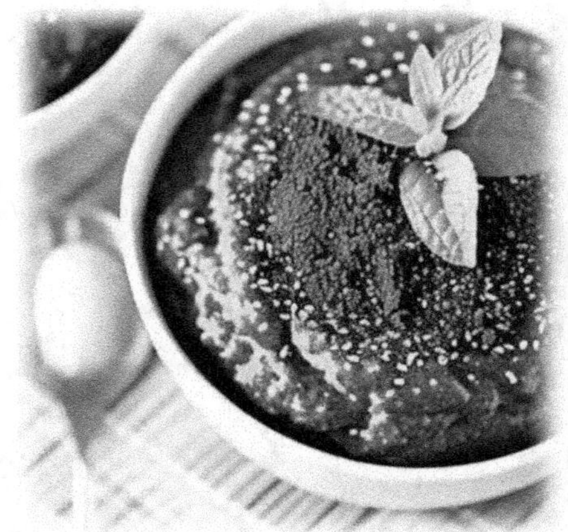

2. Cover the bowl and refrigerate for at least 2 hours or until the mixture thickens.

3. Remove from the refrigerator and stir in the shredded coconut.

4. Divide the pudding among 4 individual serving dishes.

5. Sprinkle the top of each pudding with ground cinnamon (optional).

6. Serve chilled. Enjoy!

7.Fruit Parfait

Ingredients:

- ❖ 1 cup diced fresh strawberries
- ❖ 1 cup diced fresh pineapple
- ❖ 1 cup diced fresh kiwi
- ❖ 1/2 cup low-fat plain Greek yogurt
- ❖ 1/4 cup low-sugar granola

Instructions:

1. In a medium-sized bowl, combine the diced strawberries, pineapple, and kiwi.

2. In another small bowl, mix together the yogurt and granola.

3. Layer the fruit and yogurt mixture in four individual parfait glasses.

4. Top each parfait glass with an equal amount of the granola-yogurt mixture.

5. Enjoy!

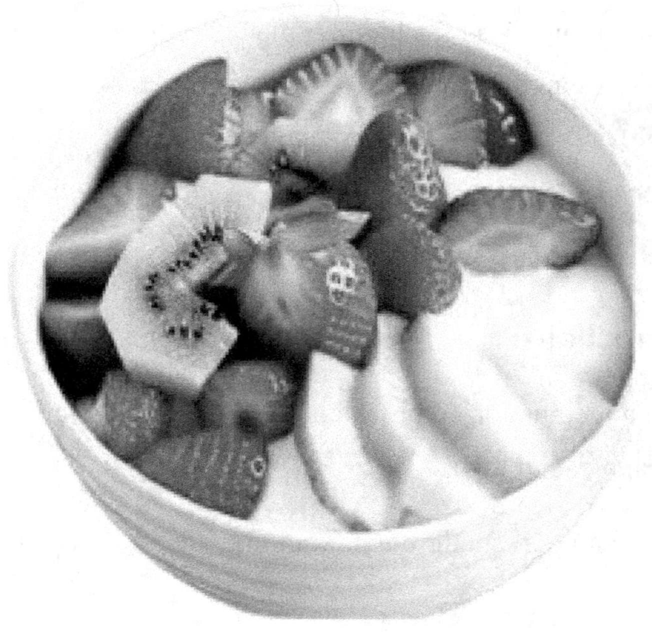

8.No Bake Chocolate Peanut Butter Oatmeal Cookies

Ingredients:

- ❖ 1/2 cup creamy peanut butter
- ❖ 1/4 cup honey
- ❖ 1/4 cup unsweetened cocoa powder
- ❖ 1/2 teaspoon pure vanilla extract
- ❖ 1/4 teaspoon ground cinnamon
- ❖ 2 cups quick-cooking oats

Instructions:

1. In a medium bowl, stir together the peanut butter, honey, cocoa powder, vanilla extract and cinnamon until fully combined.

2. Add the oats and stir until everything is evenly combined.

3. Grease a baking sheet with cooking spray.

4. Using a tablespoon, scoop out the mixture and form into balls. Place them on the baking sheet and flatten with the back of a spoon.

5. Refrigerate for at least 30 minutes before serving.

Enjoy!

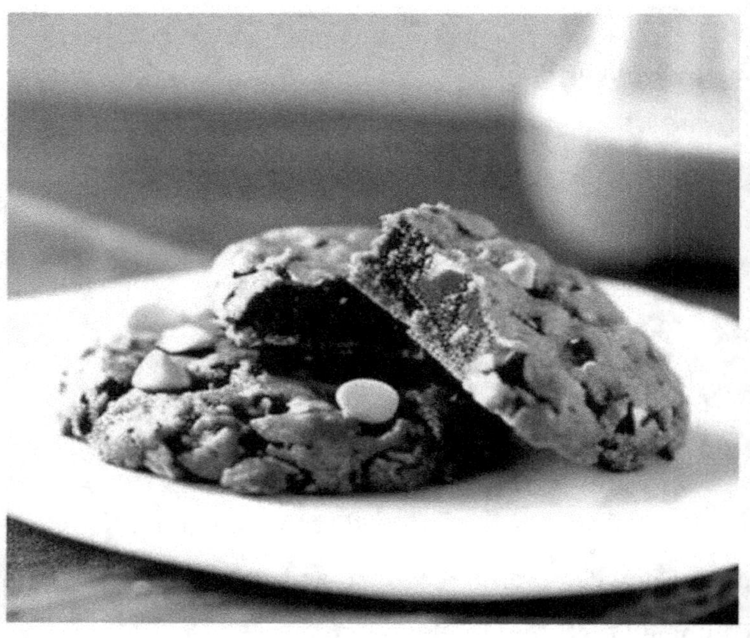

9.Vegan Chocolate Chip Cookie Dough Bites

Ingredients:

• 2 cups almond flour

• ½ cup coconut sugar

• ½ teaspoon baking soda

• ¼ teaspoon sea salt

• ¼ cup melted coconut oil

• 2 tablespoons almond milk

• 1 teaspoon vanilla extract

• ¾ cup vegan chocolate chips

Instructions:

1. Preheat oven to 350 degrees Fahrenheit.

2. In a large bowl, mix together almond flour, coconut sugar, baking soda, and salt.

3. In a separate bowl, mix together the melted coconut oil, almond milk, and vanilla extract.

4. Add the wet ingredients to the dry ingredients and mix until combined.

5. Fold in the vegan chocolate chips.

6. Line a baking sheet with parchment paper.

7. Using a tablespoon, scoop out the cookie dough and place onto the parchment paper.

8. Bake for 8-10 minutes or until golden brown.

9. Allow the cookie dough bites to cool before serving. Enjoy!

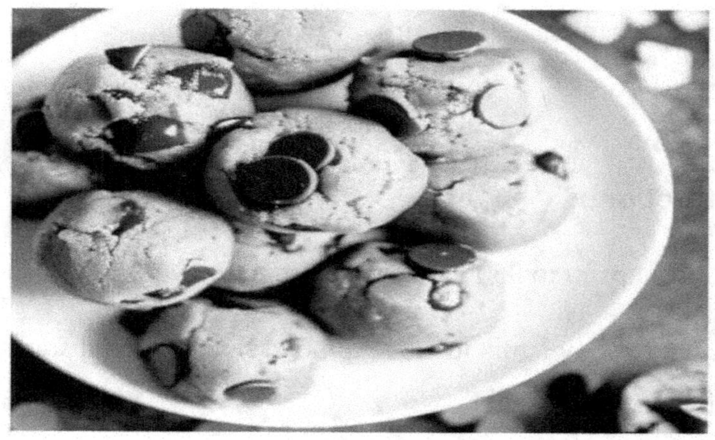

10.Chocolate Mousse with Fruit

Ingredients:

- 2 cups of frozen whipped topping, thawed
- 1/2 cup of sugar-free chocolate pudding mix
- 1/4 cup of low-fat milk
- 1/2 cup of fresh berries or other fruit of your choice
- 1/4 cup of shaved dark chocolate

Instructions:

1. In a medium bowl, whisk together the pudding mix and milk until the mix is completely dissolved.

2. Gently fold in the thawed whipped topping until combined.

3. Divide the mixture into four small glasses or dessert cups.

4. Refrigerate for at least 1 hour or until firm.

5. Top each mousse with fresh berries, shaved dark chocolate, and any other desired toppings.

6. Serve and enjoy!

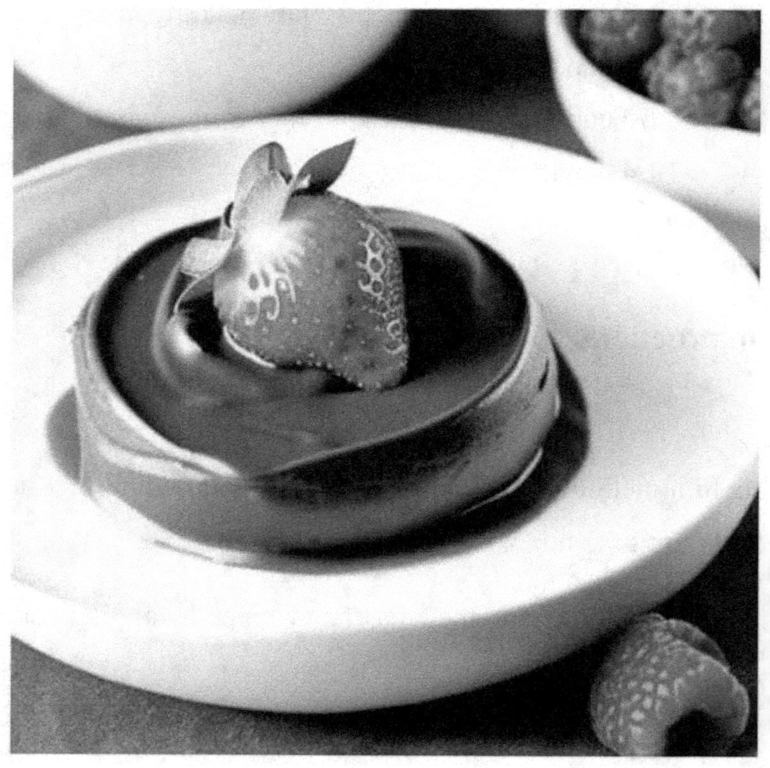

Conclusion

The Kids on a Cancer Diet cookbook has provided a wide range of delicious and nutritious recipes for children living with cancer. The recipes are designed to help children maintain a healthy diet that meets their nutritional needs, while also providing them with delicious meals that they can enjoy. The recipes also provide parents with a variety of options that are both healthy and easy to make.

This cookbook is an invaluable resource for children and families living with cancer. It provides options that are both delicious and nutritious, while also providing helpful information on nutrition, meal planning, and food safety. It is a valuable resource for families looking to create a healthy and delicious diet for their children living with cancer.

In conclusion, the Kids on a Cancer Diet cookbook is a great resource for families living with cancer. It provides a wide range of delicious and nutritious recipes for children, as well as helpful information on nutrition, meal planning, and food safety. This cookbook is an invaluable resource for families looking to create a healthy and delicious diet for their children living with cancer.

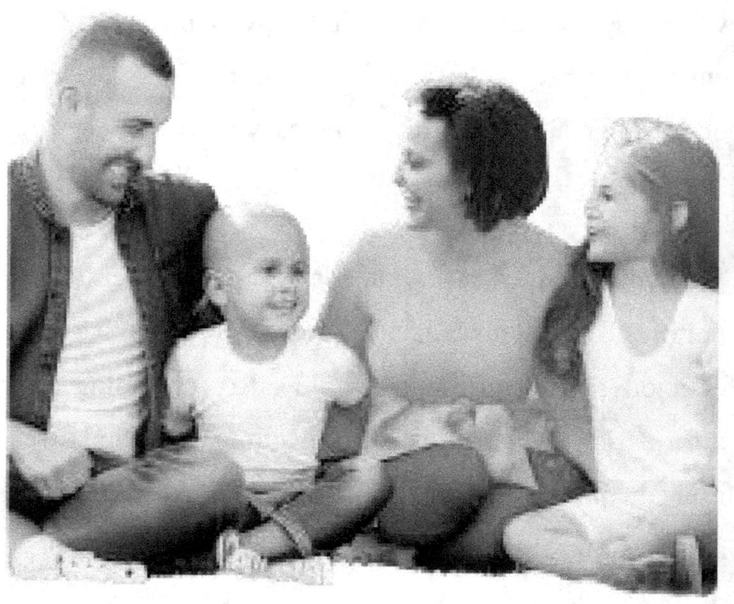

www.ingramcontent.com/pod-product-compliance
Lightning Source LLC
Chambersburg PA
CBHW061602250726
48657CB00017B/1387